Chronic Autoimmune Epithelitis - Sjogren's Syndrome and Other Autoimmune Diseases of the Exocrine Glands

Edited by Maria Maślińska

Published in London, United Kingdom

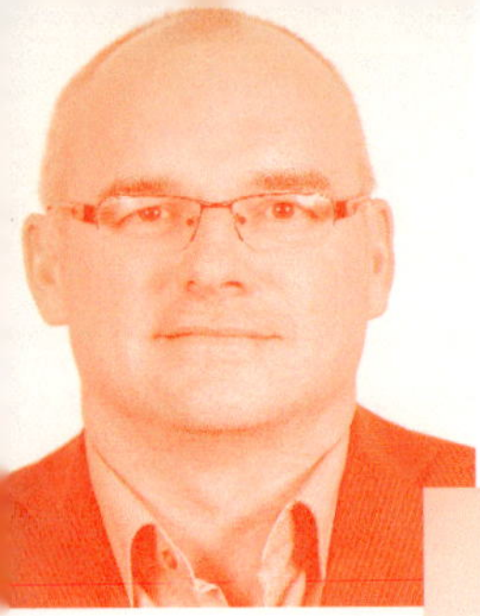
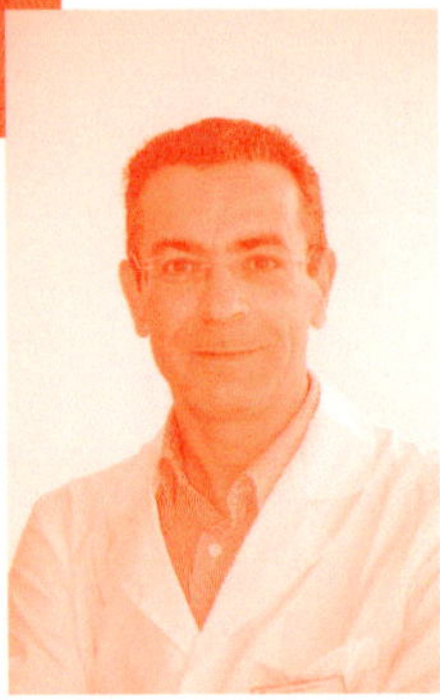
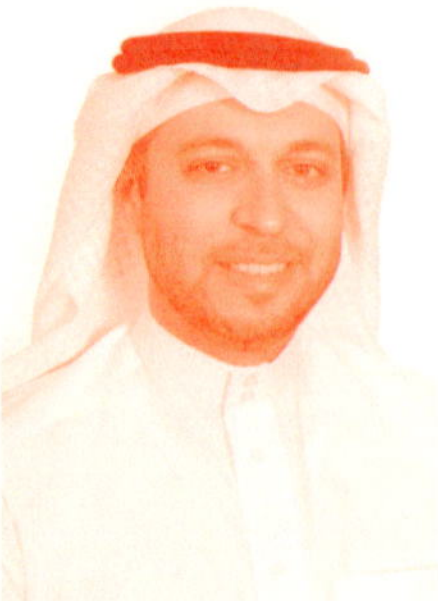
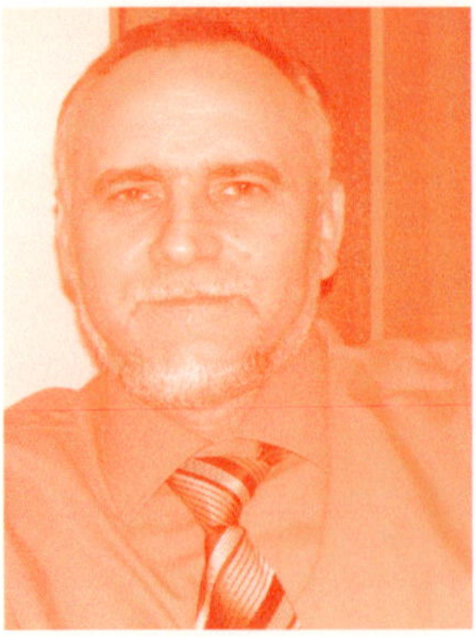
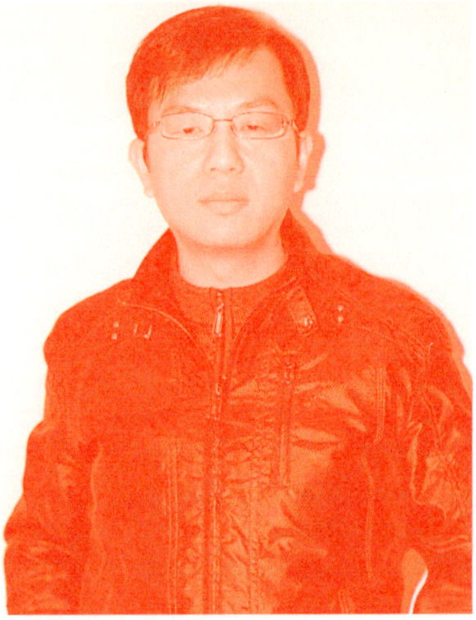
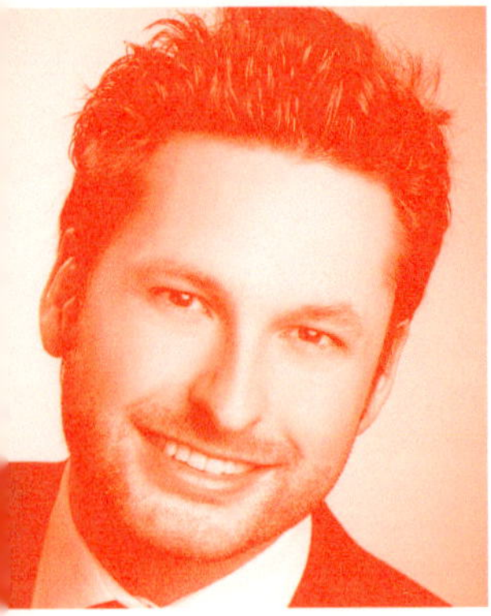
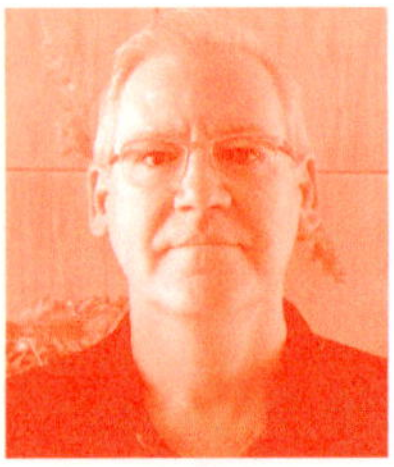

IntechOpen

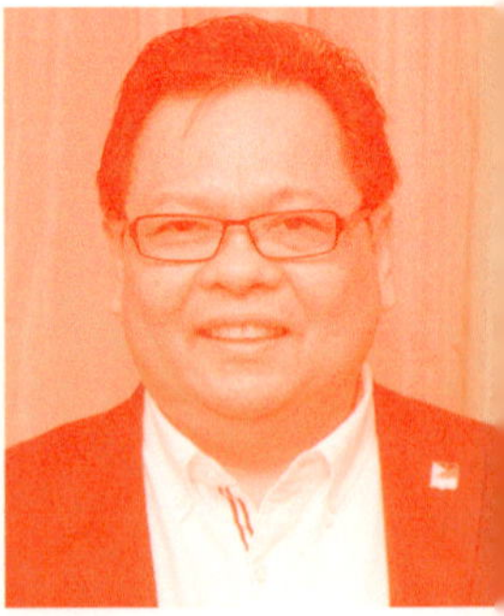
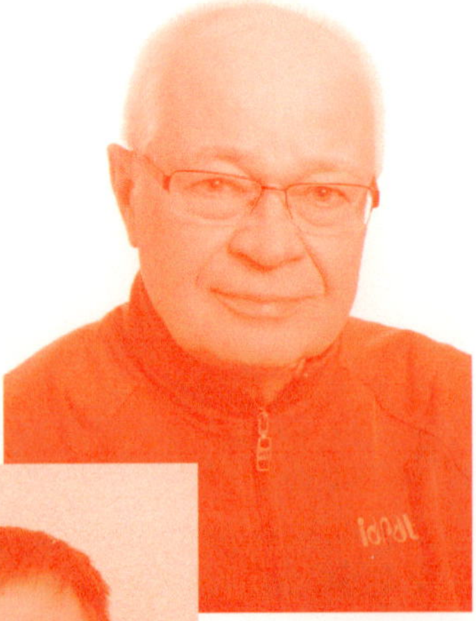
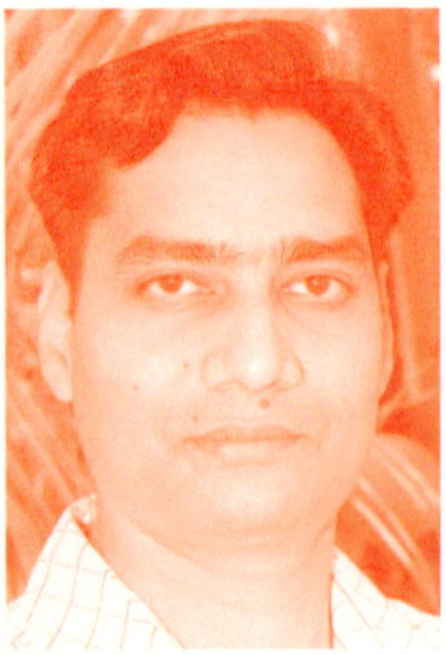
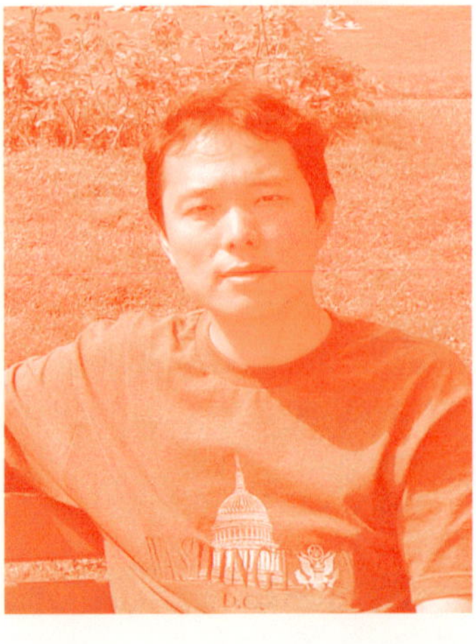
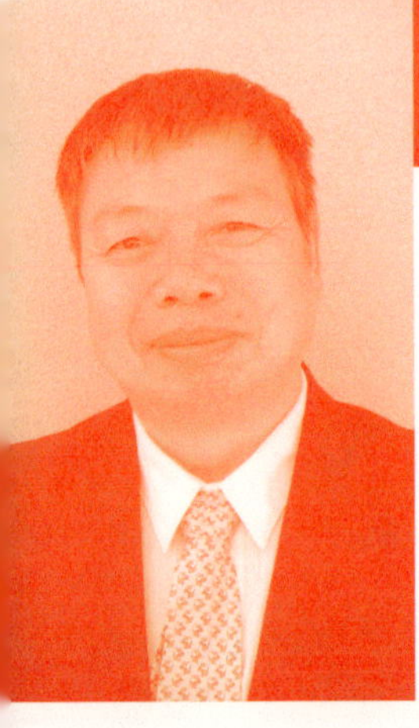
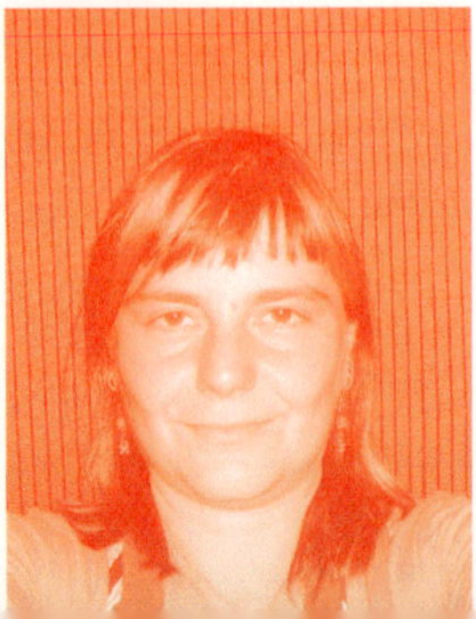

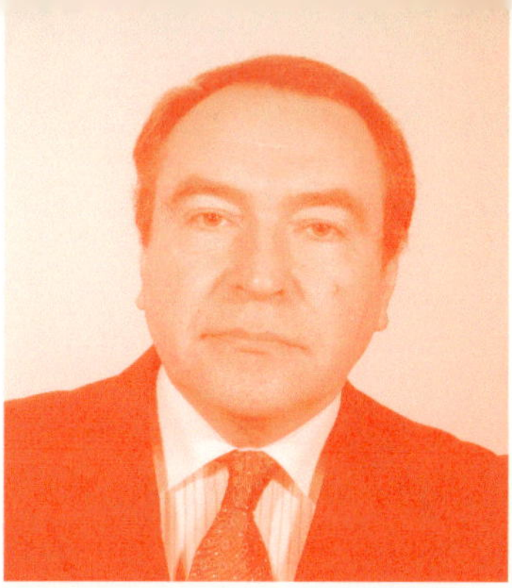
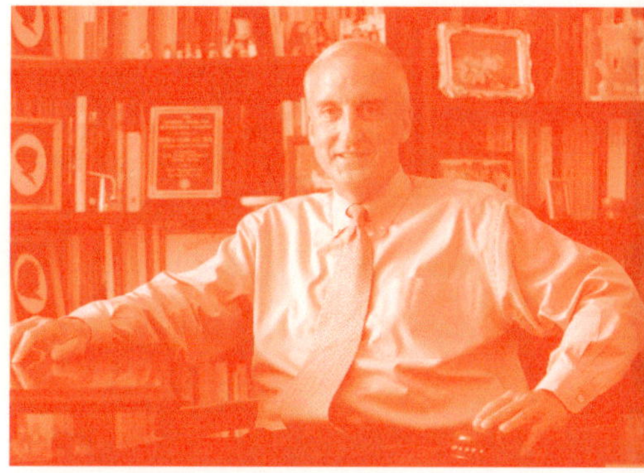
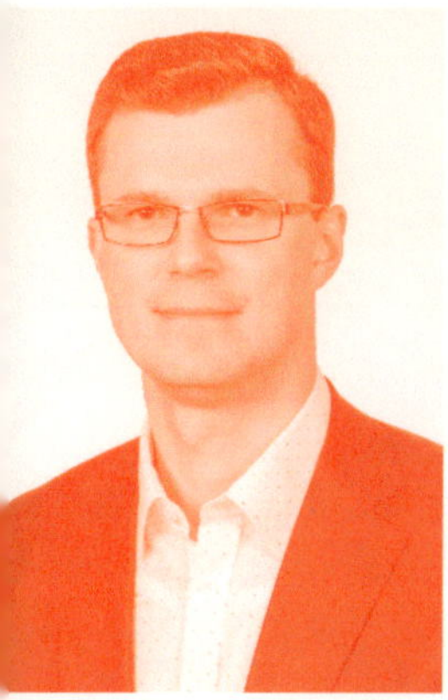
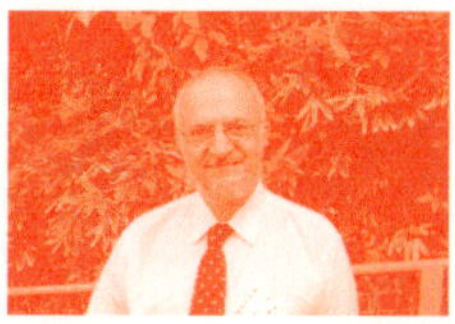
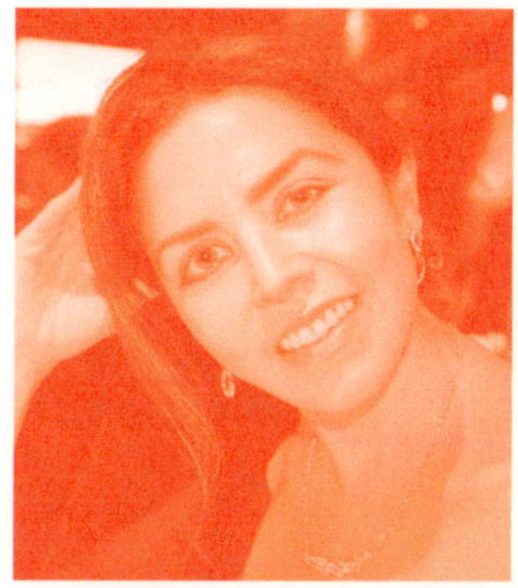

Supporting open minds since 2005

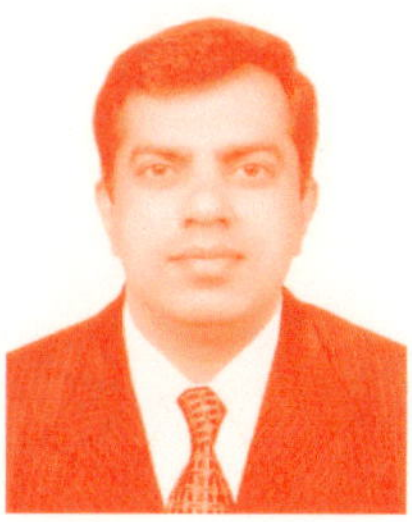
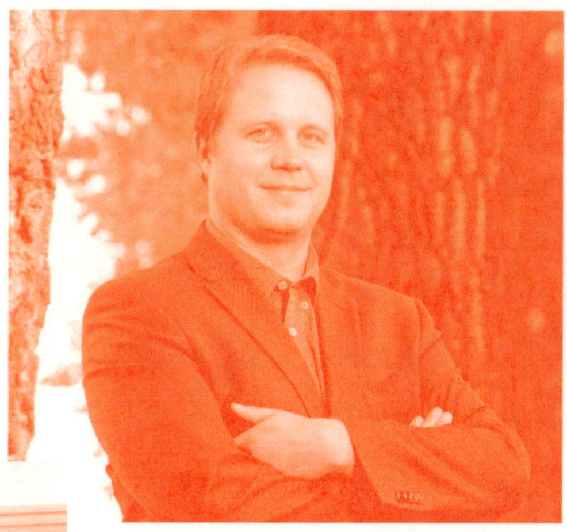
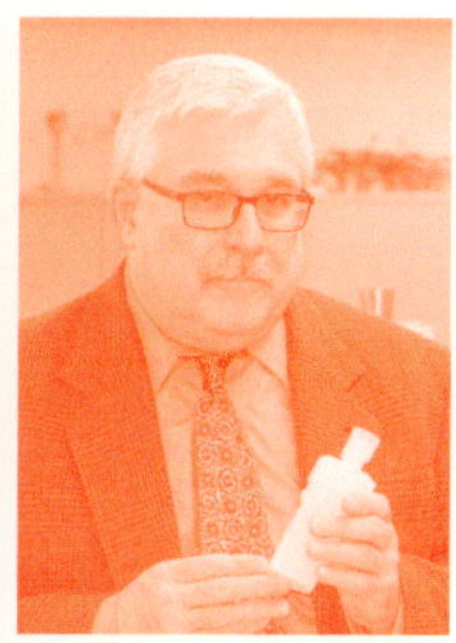
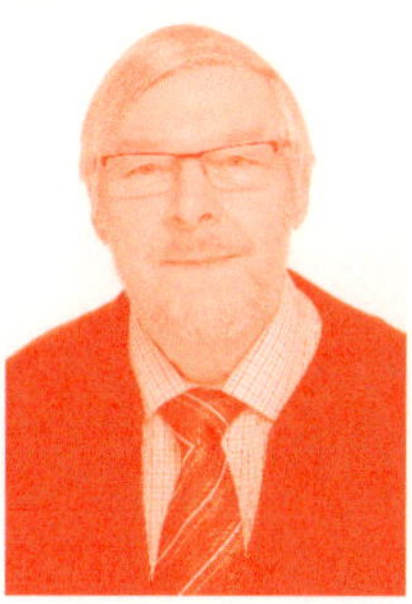
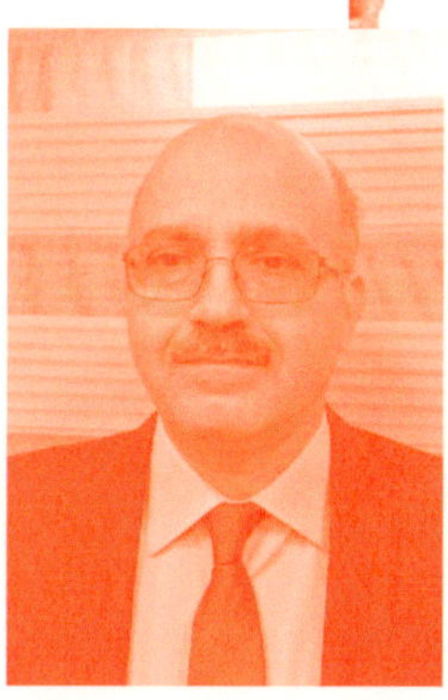
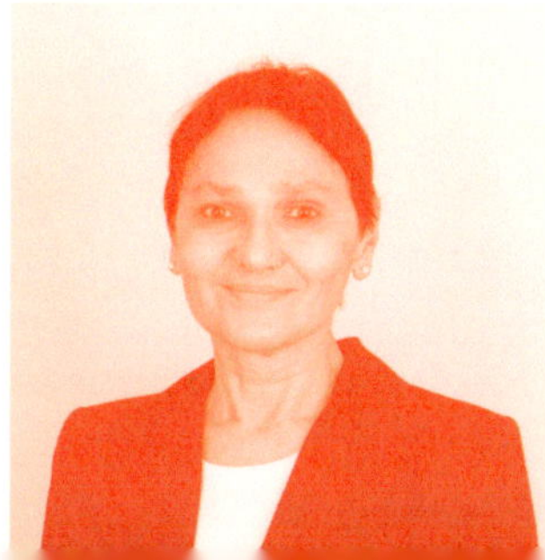
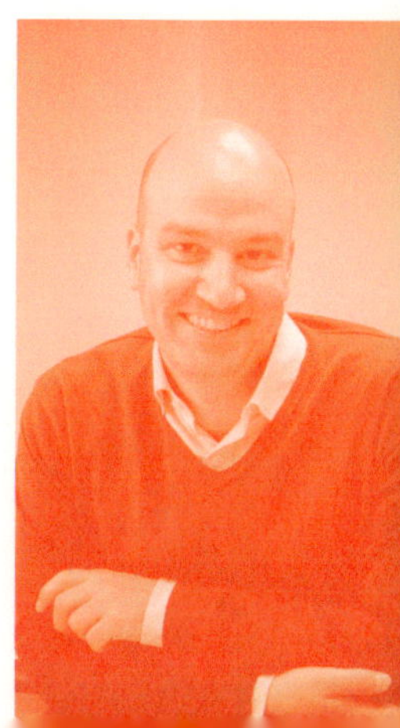

Chronic Autoimmune Epithelitis - Sjogren's Syndrome and Other Autoimmune Diseases
of the Exocrine Glands
http://dx.doi.org/10.5772/intechopen.73892
Edited by Maria Maślińska

Part of IntechOpen Book Series: Rheumatology, Volume 3
Book Series Editor: Maria Maślińska

Contributors
Agata Sebastian, Piotr Donizy, Piotr Wiland, Dorota Kopacz, Piotr Maciejewicz, Alpaslan Gokcimen, Zoltan Berger, Carla Mancilla, Bartłomiej Kamiński, Katarzyna Błochowiak, Maria Maślińska

First published in London, United Kingdom, 2019 by IntechOpen
IntechOpen is the global imprint of INTECHOPEN LIMITED, registered in England and Wales, registration number: 11086078, The Shard, 25th floor, 32 London Bridge Street
London, SE19SG - United Kingdom
Printed in Croatia

British Library Cataloguing-in-Publication Data
A catalogue record for this book is available from the British Library

Additional hard and PDF copies can be obtained from orders@intechopen.com

Chronic Autoimmune Epithelitis - Sjogren's Syndrome and Other Autoimmune Diseases
of the Exocrine Glands
Edited by Maria Maślińska
p. cm.
Print ISBN 978-1-78985-211-0
Online ISBN 978-1-78985-212-7
eBook (PDF) ISBN 978-1-78985-415-2
ISSN 2631-9233

For EU product safety concerns:
IN TECH d.o.o., Prolaz Marije Krucifikse Kozulić 3, 51000 Rijeka, Croatia,
info@intechopen.com or visit our website at intechopen.com.

IntechOpen Book Series
Rheumatology
Volume 3

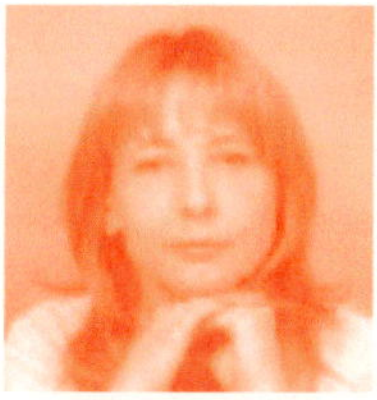

Maria Maślińska, MD, PhD, is a graduate of the 1st Medical Faculty of Warsaw Medical University (formerly Warsaw Medical Academy). She has a PhD in Medical Science from the National Institute of Geriatrics, Rheumatology and Rehabilitation in Warsaw. Maria is the deputy head of the Early Arthritis Clinic of the National Institute of Geriatrics, Rheumatology and Rehabilitation in Warsaw and the deputy editor-in-chief of the *Reumatologia* journal. Her research projects include unclassified arthritis, spondyloarthropathies, and the influence of B cells on the clinical picture of primary Sjögren's disease, including immunohistochemical and serological assessment and the profile of cytokines regulating the activity of these cells.
She has been awarded the Third Degree Group Award of the Rector of the Medical University of Warsaw for scientific achievements in the field of research related to the pathomechanism of inflammation.
Maria is a member of the Polish Society for Rheumatology and the Polish Union of Physician-Writers; author and coauthor of scientific publications, articles, and book chapters; and a lecturer at numerous courses, seminars, and conferences for general practitioners and rheumatologists.

Book Series Editor and Editor of Volume 3:
Maria Maślińska
National Institute of Geriatrics, Rheumatology and Rehabilitation
Early Arthritis Clinic, Warsaw, Poland

Scope of the Series

This book series presents new concepts of pathogenesis, including genetic, epigenetic determinants and epidemiology of rheumatic diseases. It focuses on current classification criteria, recommendations for the diagnosis and treatment of rheumatic diseases. The goal of the series is to explain various aspects of disorders associated with impaired immune response and autoimmunity processes. It also discusses risk factors associated with the development of autoimmune diseases, as well as latest discoveries and future perspectives of this extremely dynamic field of internal medicine - rheumatology.

Contents

Preface

Primary Sjögren's syndrome (pSS) is a chronic autoimmune disease associated primarily with symptoms of the eye and mouth dryness. In the literature, the term "autoimmune epithelitis" is also used to describe this disease, drawing attention to the central role of the epithelial cells in its pathogenesis.

Although exocrine glands are the main target of pSS, epithelial tissue, which constitutes a component of other organs such as kidneys, liver, lungs, or biliary ducts, is also affected, which leads to various extraglandular manifestations of the disease. The autoimmune process, which underlies the pathogenesis of pSS through the overstimulation of B cells, results in an increased risk of the development of lymphomas. Diagnosis of pSS is often very distant in time from the emergence of this condition, while effects of the long-term autoimmune processes taking place meanwhile can be irreversible.

The classification criteria of pSS were modified in recent years, in particular in light of the expanding knowledge of immunology and because of the separate group of Ig-G4-related diseases. Diagnosis of pSS must be established taking into account other epithelial autoimmune diseases, such as primary biliary cholangitis, which may coexist with pSS or occur independently mimicking pSS symptoms.

The aim of this book is to present pSS as a complex disease entity, as well as to present other autoimmune diseases in which the autoimmunity affects mainly epithelial cells and exocrine glands. The book combines the expertise of specialists in different fields of medicine—ophthalmologists, laryngologists, rheumatologists—to discuss various problems associated with Sjögren's syndrome and other autoimmune diseases with autoimmune epithelitis.

Dr. Maria Maślińska
National Institute of Geriatrics, Rheumatology and Rehabilitation,
Early Arthritis Clinic,
Warsaw, Poland

Section 1

Interdisciplinary Aspects of Primary Sjogren's Syndrome

Chapter 1

Introductory Chapter: Autoimmune Epithelitis - Discussion about Sjögren's Syndrome and Primary Biliary Cholangitis

Maria Maślińska

1. Introduction

Epithelial tissue constitutes a barrier between organs and the environment. The epithelium lines external surfaces of internal organs and inner surfaces of the walls of blood vessels. It is also a tissue that exocrine and endocrine glands consist of.

As they separate the organism from the outer environment, the epithelial structures form the first line of defense against external factors but, at the same time, an entry gate for them influencing the development of the body's microbiome and autoimmune diseases, which are associated with the disorders of microbiome composition (dysbiosis) [1, 2]. The epithelium, also as a target for viruses, interacts with the invading pathogens and is actively involved in immune response, whose course depends on particular genetic and epigenetic conditions.

Epithelial cells are often subject to apoptosis, which makes them an important source of autoantigens. Moreover, in many autoimmune diseases, epithelial cells are damaged, which leads to further release and exposition of autoantigens, with the epithelium being subject to the immune response. For example, thyrocytes are responsible for providing the main immunogens (e.g., thyroglobulin, thyroid peroxidase, TSH receptor) in autoimmune thyroiditis [3], synoviocytes are a source of cyclic citrullinated peptides in rheumatoid arthritis, and oligodendrocytes in multiple sclerosis or pancreatic endocrine glandular epithelium (beta-cells) in type 1 diabetes are a source among others of proinsulin or glutamic acid decarboxylase [4]. Hence the suggestion puts forward that autoimmune diseases could be otherwise classified as the autoimmune inflammation of the epithelium [5]. However, there are autoimmune diseases which, due to their effect on the exocrine glands, are particularly associated with epithelial damage and an autoimmune process, the primary Sjögren's syndrome (pSS) among them. The primary Sjögren's syndrome is an autoimmune disease in which the exocrine glandular epithelium is a main source of autoantigens—such as Ro/SS-A and La/SS-B ribonucleoproteins [6]. Quite often pSS may coexist with another autoimmune disorder—a primary biliary cholangitis (PBC). In PBC the epithelium (biliary epithelial cells of small bile duct) is the starting point of the autoimmune process [7]. The pathogenesis of both diseases is similar, with the significant role of epithelial cell apoptosis. **Table 1** presents the immunological and main clinical features of pSS and PBC.

 IntechOpen

The Sjögren's syndrome is an example of the development of an autoimmune epithelitis and consequences of such a process. The impact of environmental factors on the genetically susceptible subject is vital for the development of pSS. There are multiple genes (e.g., HLA-B8, HLA-Dw3, HLA-DR3, and DRw52) responsible for the individual's susceptibility to the pSS development. Particular attention has been paid to the genes for interferon regulatory factor 5 (IRF5), signal transducer and activator of transcription 4 (STAT4) in the type I interferon (IFN) system, and B lymphocyte kinase (BLK) involved in B-cell activation, which are considered as risk loci in pSS development [10]. Additionally it has been recently revealed that also epigenetic mechanisms, such as DNA methylation, histone modifications, and noncoding RNAs, may influence expression of the involved genes in autoimmune diseases, including pSS [11].

The pSS development is associated with the infection with viruses, which mainly target B cells or display tropism to lacrimal and salivary glands. Such a strong association has been confirmed in case of the Epstein–Barr virus, as well as other viruses: *Cytomegalovirus*, herpes simplex virus, and hepatitis C virus [12].

Primary Sjögren's syndrome	Primary biliary cholangitis
Exocrine glands	Liver
Chronic autoimmune disease	Chronic autoimmune disease
Anti–SS-A and anti–SS-B antibodies	Anti-mitochondrial antibodies (AMA)
ANA antibodies	ANA antibodies may be present
Exocrine glandular epithelium	Biliary epithelial cells
Predominance of CD4+ infiltrate around the salivary duct	Granuloma and predominance of CD4+ infiltrate around the bile duct
Woman > men	Woman > men
Fifth decade of life	Fifth decade of life
Primary/secondary to other autoimmune diseases	Primary/secondary to other autoimmune diseases
Genetic factors—variability in genetic factors	Genetic factors—predominant role
Infectious initiating factors: *Herpesviridae* particularly Epstein–Barr virus, CMV, herpes	Infectious initiating factors: *Escherichia coli*, *Helicobacter pylori* EBV
Symptoms of eye and mouth dryness Extraglandular manifestations (organ impairment, vasculitis, neuropathy)	Fatigue, pruritus, skin hyperpigmentation, hepatosplenomegaly Liver cirrhosis (late stage with ascites, jaundice, hepatic encephalopathy, upper digestive bleeding)
Lymphoma	Hepatocellular carcinoma
EULAR/ACR criteria for diagnosis (2016) 1. Labial salivary gland biopsy (focal lymphocytic sialadenitis) FS ≥ 1 3 points 2. Anti–SS-A/Ro positivity 3 points 3. OSS ≥5 (or van Bijsterveld score ≥ 4 1 point Schirmer's test ≤5 mm/5 min 1 point 4. Unstimulated salivary flow ≤0.1 mL/min 1 point Diagnosis ≥4 point Exclusions:	**Diagnostic criteria for PBC** 1. Elevated alkaline level of >2× ULN or elevated gamma-glutamyltransferase level of >5× ULN 2. Positivity for AMA antibodies 3. Chronic granulomatous cholangitis at liver biopsy Diagnosis presence of at least two of the three criteria

ULN, upper limit of normal.

Table 1.
The immunological and main clinical features of pSS and PBC [8, 9].

The epithelitis in pSS starts with an influence of certain external factors, such as viruses, rare bacteria, or ultraviolet radiation on epithelial cells. This leads to cell apoptosis and expression of autoantigens (SS-A and SS-B ribonucleoproteins), which are presented to autoreactive T cells. As it is recently highlighted in the literature, endothelial cells have, therefore, antigen presentation properties, although this is not their main feature, as it is the case with antigen-presenting cells (APCs), such as dendritic cells, macrophages, and B cells. Also salivary gland epithelial cells (SGEC) express MHC class I and MHC class II (HLA-DR) molecules and functional co-stimulator B7.1 (CD80) and B7.2 (CD86) molecules and may transmit signals to T lymphocytes as nonprofessional APCs [13, 14].

Other processes responsible for the development at this stage include the activation of the innate immune system, with the activation of Toll-like receptors (especially TLR3, TLR7, TLR9) and the production of interferon alpha (IFN-α) by plasma dendritic cells (pDCs) stimulating epithelial cells, dendritic cells, and neutrophils for the production of the B-cell stimulating factor and APRIL [15]. There are infiltrates in the exocrine glands initially composed mainly of T cells, whereas the activation of B lymphocytes by growth factors, such as BAFF and APRIL, results in hypergammaglobulinemia and the production of anti–SS-A and anti–SS-B autoantibodies as a secondary immune response. B cells and macrophages also produce proinflammatory cytokines, chemokines, and adhesion molecules.

The disease starts with the epithelial inflammation and impaired function of the exocrine glands manifesting themselves, for example, in the enlargement of the glands and reduction of the secretion of saliva or tears. It evolves then into the phase of systemic disease with the organ involvement and general manifestations (fever, weight loss, fatigue). Although the Sjögren's syndrome is most often associated with the functional impairment of lacrimal and salivary glands (symptoms included in the current criteria of diagnosis [16]), it also affects glands of the digestive system, pancreas, liver, gall bladder, respiratory glands, and even sweat glands. Their function is impaired through the reduction of secretion of the aqueous phase and changes in density of the secretion, leading to the emergence of various clinical features: from the feeling of mouth or eye dryness, through recurrent cholelithiasis and nephrolithiasis, to stones in the salivary glands.

The consequence of the involvement of epithelia in pSS and its damage is the emergence of the way of entry for pathogens in the alimentary tract (from the oral cavity to the rectum), as well as in the respiratory tract. In the case of imbalance of the microbiome and the occurrence of dysbiosis, also commensals, which become potential pathogens in such circumstances, may cross the damaged epithelial barrier. Proteins from the epithelial cells of the mouth, intestines, and skin, as well as bacterial (commensal) proteins, may initiate an immune response to Ro60 (theory of Ro60-reactive B cells) and activation of T cells, as consequence of molecular mimicry [17]. The role of fungal (*Candida*) infections in pSS development was also studied, revealing there was no significant relationship between *Candida albicans* and the rate and amount of salivary secretion, although such relationship was found in pathogenic species, such as *C. tropicalis*, *C. glabrata*, and *C. krusei* [18].

In **Table 2** the main clinical manifestations of pSS resulting from the epithelial damage are presented.

What is particularly important, continuous stimulation of B lymphocytes by activating agents, primarily BAFF and APRIL, causes germinal center (GC) formation and the formation of secondary lymphoid tissue, which in turn leads to the increased risk of lymphoma development. The most common lymphoma emerging in the course of pSS is the marginal zone B-cell lymphoma (MZBCL), the mucosa-associated lymphoid tissue (MALT) type being predominant. The diffuse large B-cell lymphoma (DLBCL), rare T-cell lymphoma, or NK-cell lymphoma are

Localization	Effect
Nasal and oral cavity	Oral candidiasis, dental caries, periodontitis otitis media, dry nose, chronic sinusitis, nasal bleeding, weakening of the sense of smell
Bronchi	Difficulty in swallowing, dry cough, hoarseness, recurrent bronchitis and less frequent bronchioles, bronchial hyperresponsiveness and accompanying dry cough, infections
Lungs	Interstitial lung disease
Stomach	Chronic gastritis, malabsorption, susceptibility to *H. pylori* infection
Gut	Celiac disease, colitis Gluten sensitivity [19, 20]
Liver	Hepatitis, cholangitis
Pancreas	Pancreatitis
Kidneys and urine tract	Interstitial nephritis with distal renal tubular acidosis (dRTA). Glomerulonephritis with coexisting cryoglobulinemia and urolithiasis

Table 2.
The main clinical manifestations of pSS due to the epithelial damage.

less common. The occurrence of MZBCL has been observed in about 8% of pSS patients; it is 40 times higher than in the healthy population [21, 22].

2. Focusing on MALT lymphoma

The most important feature of MALT lymphoma is the presence of neoplastic cells (mainly B cells, as well as T cells) within epithelial structures, which may lead to destruction of the glandular architecture, also because of the formation of solid infiltrations.

Lymphomas in pSS are predominantly localized in salivary glands, which has been confirmed in many studies [23], whereas in the general population, MALT lymphoma is most often located in the stomach. The occurrence of MALT lymphoma in the stomach is proven to be associated with *H. pylori* infection [24]. The primary division of MALT lymphomas depending on the location is shown in **Table 3**.

Subtypes of lymphoma due to localization		
MALT	NALT	Nasopharynx-associated lymphoid tissue
	BALT	Bronchus-associated lymphoid tissue
	LALT	Larynx-associated lymphoid tissue
	GALT	Gut-associated lymphoid tissue
SALT	Skin-associated lymphoid tissue	
CALT	Conjunctiva-associated lymphoid tissue	
SDALT	Salivary duct-associated lymphoid tissue	
O-MALT	Organized mucosa-associated lymphatic tissue-specific type of MALT affecting Waldeyer's tonsillar ring	
D-MALT	Diffuse mucosa-associated lymphatic tissue-specific type of the disease, cells not organized into a separate macroscopically and anatomically identifiable mass, but spread throughout the mucosa of different organs	

Table 3.
Division due to the localization of MALT lymphoma [22, 25].

3. Sjögren's syndrome and primary biliary cholangitis as autoimmune epithelitis: general rules for treatment

3.1 The treatment of primary Sjögren's syndrome involves a dual approach

- A topical treatment, which aims to protect the epithelial barrier of the eye, oral cavity, and vagina

- Inhibition of organ changes, as well as the elimination of general symptoms, such as fatigue, fever, malaise, or lymphadenopathy [26, 27]

3.1.1 Topical treatment

1. Oral cavity

   A. Saliva substitutes: hydroxymethylcellulose-containing oral spray, proper hydration by consuming more liquids, and regularly rinsing the mouth

The stimulation of salivary flow, obtained with the use of pilocarpine or cevimeline, parasympathomimetics, and muscarinic agonists affecting M1 and M3 receptors, after considering possible contraindications for their use.

Antifungal and antimicrobial treatment with medications such as chlorhexidine; the use of nonfluoride remineralizing agents as concomitant therapy.

Diet modification is recommended: eating slightly acidic products such as lemon, supplementing diet with unsaturated fatty acids (omega-3), and avoiding sweets and sweet effervescent beverages.

Quitting smoking is strongly recommended.

2. Dry eye

   A. The modification of environmental factors, which may increase the dry eye symptoms, such as air condition, exposure to dust, and prolonged work at computer screen.

When possible, the discontinuation of treatment with medications resulting in the reduction of tears or disruption of their composition.

Artificial tears, gels, ointments, special contact lenses, topical autologous serum, and special contact lenses.

Punctual plugs (temporary or permanent).

The eyelid therapy: massages and warm compresses.

The eyelid surgery (e.g., blepharoplasty).

Topical immunosuppression: steroids and cyclosporine A.

3. Vaginal dryness

   Vaginal dryness treatment is based on the use of intimate moisturizers and sexual lubricants and pH balance stabilizers free from hormones and skin irritants. In some cases the use of estrogen topical medication may be found useful.

3.1.2 General treatment

Immunosuppressive drugs such as azathioprine, methotrexate, leflunomide, mycophenolic acid, cyclosporine A (topical, rare oral), and cyclophosphamide effects are used to inhibit general symptoms and organ involvement [26, 27].

Among biological drugs, rituximab (anti-CD20 monoclonal antibody) has been showing positive results in current clinical trials and is used to inhibit certain aspects of the disease. Rituximab improves saliva flow rate and lacrimal gland function (discussed), diminishes fatigue and malaise, and is recommended in case of cryoglobulinemia or vasculitis-related peripheral nervous system involvement or other severe neurologic manifestations of this disease.

Glucocorticosteroids (GCS) are used in immunosuppressive therapy combined with other immunosuppressive drugs. Pulses of GCS are used in the case of the intensification of organ changes, vasculitis, and nervous system involvement.

Intravenous immunoglobulin administration and plasma exchanges are used in life-threatening cases of nervous system involvement and vasculitis.

Other: Vitamin D supplementation and aerobic exercises are recommended.

3.2 Treatment of primary biliary cholangitis

3.2.1 Treatment for itching

Antihistamines, e.g., loratadine or diphenhydramine, are used. Cholestyramine as the addition to beverages and foods may be used. Rifampicin, an antibiotic which may act as a medicine against itching, may also be administered [28]. Opioid antagonists containing naloxone or naltrexone inhibit pruritus by their effects on the central nervous system [29].

3.3 Treatment for dry eyes and mouth as in pSS

3.3.1 General treatment

Ursodeoxycholic acid (UDCA) is the main medication used in biliary cholangitis. A complementary therapy with obeticholic acid was introduced in 2016, as second-line treatment. If the UDCA treatment is ineffective, the use of fibrates (e.g., bezafibrate) in combination therapy (UDCA plus fibrate) is also considered; ongoing clinical trials have yielded encouraging results [30]. Of the immunosuppressants, the use of methotrexate (MTX), as a drug which may affect pruritus score, serum level of alkaline phosphatase, or IgM level, is discussed [31], although there were observations that MTX could increase mortality in this group of patients [32]. There were clinical trials with rituximab [33] and with ustekinumab [34], but at the present time, they have not produced positive results to the expected extent. The liver transplant aims at prolonging the patient's life, but it is reported that up to 29% of patients develop a relapse of the disease in the transplanted organ [35]. Therefore, the use of UDCA after transplantation is still recommended.

3.3.2 Changes in the style of life

PBC is a chronic autoimmune liver disease in which a lifestyle is particularly important. Reducing the intake of foods with high sodium content, avoiding alcohol, as well as being careful with new medications or dietary supplements are extremely important. Physical exercise is recommended to reduce risk of bone loss and muscle weakness.

4. Conclusions

The epithelium is an important element of the human body due to its protective, secretory, and transporting functions. It is also the target for the immunological

DOI: http://dx.doi.org/10.5772/intechopen.86258

processes. The impact of environmental, genetic, and epigenetic factors, leading to the epithelial cell damage/apoptosis, may cause a breakdown of epithelium hemostasis and the development of autoimmune diseases, Sjögren's syndrome being its prominent representative. For years pSS was associated with autoimmune epithelial inflammation and referred to as the "autoimmune epithelitis." However, the spectrum of diseases related to the epithelial autoimmunity is wider including, e.g., primary biliary cholangitis. The damaged epithelium is a source of autoantigens, and a persistent immune cell stimulation may lead to the lymphomas associated with the mucosa. Adoption of a wider perspective, combining the clinical experience and scientific knowledge, in an approach to the problem of epithelitis enables making the connection between emerging symptoms and autoimmune diseases, leading to the earlier diagnosis and introduction of proper treatment. Thus the reduction in an activity of the immune process and inhibition of further damage to the epithelium and of loss of its protective properties can be achieved.

Author details

Maria Maślińska
National Institute of Geriatrics, Rheumatology and Rehabilitation, Early Arthritis Clinic, Warsaw, Poland

*Address all correspondence to: maslinskam@gmail.com

References

[1] Honda K, Littman DR. The microbiota in adaptive immune homeostasis and disease. Nature. 2016;**535**(7610):75-84

[2] Mandl T, Marsal J, Olsson P, Ohlsson B, Andréasson K. Severe intestinal dysbiosis is prevalent in primary Sjögren's syndrome and is associated with systemic disease activity. Arthritis Research & Therapy. 2017;**19**(1):237

[3] Chistiakov DA. Immunogenetics of Hashimoto's thyroiditis. Journal of Autoimmune Disease. 2005;**2**(1):1

[4] Ziegler AG, Nepom GT. Prediction and pathogenesis in type 1 diabetes. Immunity. 2010;**32**(4):468-478

[5] Mitsias D, Kapsogeorgou E, Moutsopoulos H. Sjögren's syndrome: Why autoimmune epithelitis? Oral Diseases. 2006;**12**:523-532

[6] Voulgarelis M, Tzioufas AG. Current aspects of pathogenesis in Sjögren's syndrome. Therapeutic Advances in Musculoskeletal Disease. 2010;**2**(6):325-334

[7] Webb GJ, Siminovitch KA, Hirschfield GM. The immunogenetics of primary biliary cirrhosis: A comprehensive review. Journal of Autoimmunity. 2015;**64**:42-52. DOI: 10.1016/j.jaut.2015.07.004

[8] Selmi C, Meroni PL, Gershwin ME. Primary biliary cirrhosis and Sjögren's syndrome: Autoimmune epithelitis. Journal of Autoimmunity. 2011;**39**(1-2):34-42

[9] Zhu Y, Ma X, Tang X, Hua B. Liver damage in primary biliary cirrhosis and accompanied by primary Sjögren's syndrome: A retrospective pilot study. Central-European Journal of Immunology. 2016;**41, 2**:182-187

[10] Huang XF, Cheng Q, Jiang CM, et al. The immune factors involved in the pathogenesis, diagnosis, and treatment of Sjogren's syndrome. Clinical and Developmental Immunology. 2013. Article ID 160491

[11] Imgenberg-Kreuz J, Sandling JK, Nordmark G. Epigenetic alterations in primary Sjögren's syndrome—An overview. Clinical Immunology. 2018;**196**:12-20

[12] García-Carrasco M, Fuentes-Alexandro S, Escárcega RO, et al. Pathophysiology of Sjögren's syndrome. Archives of Medical Research. 2006;**37**(8):921-932

[13] Kapsogeorgou EK, Moutsopoulos HM, Manoussakis MN. Functional expression of a costimulatory B7.2 (CD86) protein on human salivary gland epithelial cells that interacts with CD28 receptor, but has reduced binding to CTLA4. Journal of Immunology. 2001;**166**:3107-3113

[14] Matsumura R, Umemiya K, Goto T, et al. Glandular and extraglandular expression of costimulatory molecules in patients with Sjögren's syndrome. Annals of the Rheumatic Diseases. 2001;**60**:473-482

[15] Youinou P, Pers JO. Disturbance of cytokine networks in Sjögren's syndrome. Arthritis Research & Therapy. 2011;**13**:227

[16] Shiboski CH, Shiboski SC, Seror R, et al. 2016 American College of Rheumatology/European league against rheumatism classification criteria for primary Sjögren's syndrome: A consensus and data-driven methodology involving three international patient cohorts. Arthritis & Rhematology. 2016;**69**(1): 35-45. DOI: 10.1002/art.39859

[17] Szymula A, Rosenthal J, Szczerba BM, Bagavant H, Fu SM, Deshmukh US. T cell epitope mimicry between

Sjögren's syndrome antigen A (SSA)/ Ro60 and oral, gut, skin and vaginal bacteria. Clinical Immunology. 2014;**152**(1-2):1-9

[18] Cackowska-Lass A, Kochańska B, Naumiuk Ł, Samet A. Saliva secretion and prevalence of some microorganisms in the oral cavity in patients with Sjögren's syndrome. Czasopismo Stomatologiczne. 2010;**63**(2):79-89

[19] Szodoray P, Barta Z, Lakos G, Szakáll S, Zeher M. Coeliac disease in Sjögren's syndrome—A study of 111 Hungarian patients. Rheumatology International. 2004;**24**(5):278-282

[20] Lidén M, Kristjánsson G, Valtýsdóttir S, Hällgren R. Gluten sensitivity in patients with primary Sjögren's syndrome. Scandinavian Journal of Gastroenterology. 2007;**42**(8):962-967

[21] Baimpa E, Dahabreh IJ, Voulgarelis M, Moutsopoulos HM. Hematologic manifestations and predictors of lymphoma development in primary Sjögren syndrome: Clinical and pathophysiologic aspects. Medicine (Baltimore). 2009;**88**(5):284-293

[22] Hayashi D, Devenney-Cakir B, Lee JC, et al. Mucosa-associated lymphoid tissue lymphoma: Multimodality imaging and Histopathologic correlation. American Journal of Roentgenology. 2010;**195**(2):W105-W117

[23] Nocturne G, Mariette X. Sjögren syndrome-associated lymphomas: An update on pathogenesis and management. British Journal of Haematology. 2015;**168**:317-327

[24] El Miedany YM, Baddour M, Ahmed I, Fahmy H. Sjogren's syndrome: Concomitant *H. pylori* infection and possible correlation with clinical parameters. Joint, Bone, Spine. 2005;**72**:135-141

[25] Cesta MF. Normal structure, function, and histology of mucosa-associated lymphoid tissue. Toxicologic Pathology. 2006;**34**(5):599-608

[26] Ramos-Casals M, Brito-Zerón P, Sisó-Almirall A, Bosch X, Tzioufas AG. Topical and systemic medications for the treatment of primary Sjögren's syndrome. Nature Reviews Rheumatology. 2012;**8**(7):399-411

[27] P1 B-Z, Sisó-Almirall A, Bové A, Kostov BA, Ramos-Casals M. Primary Sjögren syndrome: An update on current pharmacotherapy options and future directions. Expert Opinion on Pharmacotherapy. 2013;**14**(3):279-289

[28] Khurana S, Singh P. Rifampin is safe for treatment of pruritus due to chronic cholestasis: A meta-analysis of prospective randomized-controlled trials. Liver International. 2006;**26**(8):943-948

[29] Trivedi HD, Lizaola B, Tapper EB, Bonder A. Management of Pruritus in primary biliary cholangitis: A narrative review. American Journal of Medicine. 2017;**130**:744-744.e7

[30] Corpechot C, Chazouillères O, Rousseau A. A placebo-controlled trial of bezafibrate in primary biliary cholangitis. New England Journal of Medicine. 2018;**378**:2171-2181

[31] Giljaca V, Poropat G, Stimac D, Gluud C. Methotrexate for primary biliary cirrhosis. Cochrane Database of Systematic Reviews. 2010;**5**:CD004385

[32] Gong Y, Gluud C. Methotrexate for primary biliary cirrhosis. Cochrane Database of Systematic Reviews. 2005;**3**:CD004385

[33] Tsuda M, Moritoki Y, Lian ZX, et al. Biochemical and immunologic effects of rituximab in patients with primary biliary cirrhosis and an incomplete response to ursodeoxycholic acid. Hepatology. 2012;**55**:512-521

[34] Hirschfield GM, Gershwin ME, Strauss R, et al. Ustekinumab for patients with primary biliary cholangitis who have an inadequate response to ursodeoxycholic acid: A proof-of-concept study. Hepatology. 2016;**64**:189-199

[35] Montano-Loza AJ, Bhanji RA, Wasilenko S, Mason AL. Systematic review: Recurrent autoimmune liver diseases after liver transplantation. Alimentary Pharmacology & Therapeutics. 2017;**45**:485-500. DOI: 10.1111/apt.13894

Chapter 2

Morphology of Salivary and Lacrimal Glands

Alpaslan Gokcimen

Abstract

Generally, the tissues consist of stroma and parenchyma. The epithelial tissue, which forms the basis of exocrine glands, is rich in parenchyma. The secretions of salivary glands are functionally related to the digestion, and the secretions of the lacrimal glands protect the eye surface and allow to maintain a proper vision. The parotid is a pure serous gland and consists of serous acinus. The submandibular gland is a mixed gland consisting of serous acini and mucous tubules, and the acinus is predominant. The sublingual gland is a mixed gland composed of serous acini and mucous tubules, such as the submandibular gland, but the mucous tubules are predominant. The secretions of salivary glands reach the oral cavity with the intercalated canal, the intralobular canal, the interlobular canal, and the main duct channel. "Stenon duct" in the parotid gland, "Wharton duct" in the submandibular gland, and "major sublingual" duct in the sublingual gland open into the oral cavity. The lacrimal gland is structurally similar to salivary glands. This gland was divided into lobules by irregular tight connective tissue. In the lobules, acinar cells and mucus tubules are located together.

Keywords: salivary glands, lacrimal glands, morphology, functions

1. Introduction

The smallest unit of a living organism is the cell and cells congregate to form tissues. The cells that make up the tissues do not only have similar shapes but also form a community to perform specified functions. Basically, the tissues consist of two parts: parenchyma and stroma. Stroma forms the skeleton of the structure. The parenchyma is the tissue's functional part and is located inside the stroma. Therefore, the tissue as a whole performs specific tasks and functions. In normal conditions, stroma and parenchyma are in certain ratios in each tissue. In some tissues parenchyma is predominant, as in epithelial tissue, while in a connective tissue, it makes up its minority. Basically, according to the rate of parenchyma and stroma, there are four kinds of tissues: epithelial tissue (epithelium), connective tissue, muscle tissue, and nerve tissue. In the second week of embryonic development, the bilaminar embryo disc forms, while the trilaminar embryo disc emerges at its third week. Tissues take origin from the different layers of this embryonic disc. The epithelial tissue originates from all of the embryonic germ leaves [1–3].

Ectoderm-derived epithelial structures are as follows: sweat glands and ducts, oral cavity, and vaginal and anal canal epithelium [1–3].

Mesoderm-derived epithelial structures include blood vessel endothelium, mesothelium that lines up body cavities, and epithelium covering genitourinary system and tubules [1–3].

IntechOpen

The epithelial tissue originating from endoderm is located on the inner surface of the esophagus, as an epithelium covering the stomach-intestinal tract, an epithelium surrounding the gallstones, large glandules such as in the liver and pancreas, and an epithelium located in the respiratory system [1–3].

1.1 Features of epithelial tissues

a. Basal membrane: The epithelium is never found in space but is located on the basal membrane as single or multiple layers (**Figure 1a**, **b**). All cells are arranged on the basement membrane but with the exception of ependymal cells, mesangial cells, and macula densa [4, 5].

b. Diversity: We can summarize the main function of epithelial tissue as covering, protection, secretion, and absorption. It varies according to these functional differences. The epidermis covers the outer surface of our body and protects it (**Figure 2**). The covering function protects not only the body's external surface but also the inner part of the lumen structures such as the small intestine and colon, the trachea, and the urinary system (**Figures 3–6**). The epithelial cells progress in the lower connective tissue and form different gland structures such as tubular and simple branched tubular. In this way, mucous tubules and serous acini are formed. Therefore, suitable serous, mucous, or mixed secretions are produced. These glands give out their secretions through duct channels [4, 6].

c. Polarity: The epithelium has three surfaces. These include apical, lateral, and basal surface. There are membrane extensions on the apical surface such as cilia, microvillus, flagella, and stereocilia. Microvillus is especially important for these structures in food exchange. The small intestine is the best example of it (**Figure 3**). In particular, the microvillus is located in the proximal part of the kidney where the absorption occurs (**Figure 7**). The microvillus in the epithelial cells provides reabsorption of important substances. Reabsorption is also provided by basal invaginations. Basal invaginations can be observed in the ductus striata of the salivary glands and proximal and distal tubules of the kidney at best. The substances taken with the apical surface of the epithelial cell are given to the basal part by active transport [4, 6].

d. The cilia are mobile and they are located in the respiratory system (**Figure 5**). Cilia make the sweeping movement from the trachea to the oral cavity. In this way, harmful substances such as microorganisms and carbon particles are thrown out of the body. The cilia are also found in the uterus and tuba uterina of female genital system (**Figures 8**, **9a**, **b**). Cilia in the female genital system sweep the secretion to pass the zygote from the uterus into the uterine cavity. Flagella is seen in the spermium, and it provides the spermium moves in this way (**Figure 10a**, **b**) [4–8]. Stereocilia are a non-movement structure (**Figure 11**). Stereocilia increase the surface area of the epididymis and allow absorption of testicular fluid and phagocytosis of pathological sperm. Stereocilia which reside in the hair cells of the inner ear are involved in signal generation [4–8].

The lateral surface of the epithelium, there are intercellular binding complexes: non-permeable connections, anchor connections, and gap junction. Zonula occludens are non-permeable; zonula adherens, hemidesmosomes, and desmosome are anchors; and gap junction is the intercellular connections that provide communication.

Basal invagination is present in the epithelium. These are the finger in folds that the cell membrane makes at baseline and parallel to each other; there are abundant mitochondria in these recesses. Basal invaginations are known as ductus striata of salivary gland's duct channels. Basal invaginations are also present in the epithelium

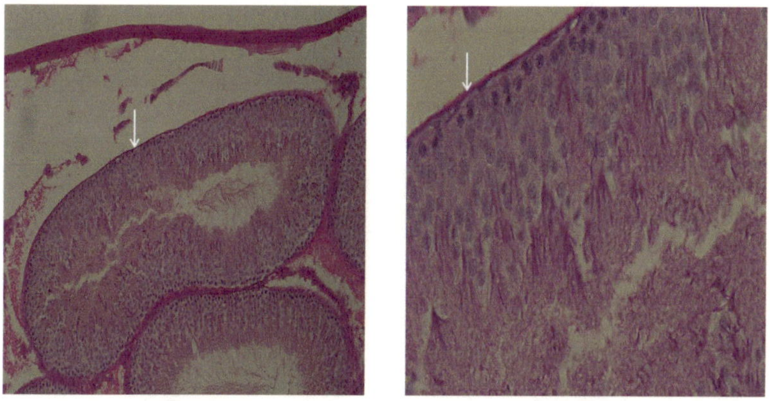

Figure 1.
(a, b) In the section taken from the testis, the basement membrane is seen as a red-pink line. Hematoxylin–eosin staining (Dr. Alpaslan Gokcimen).

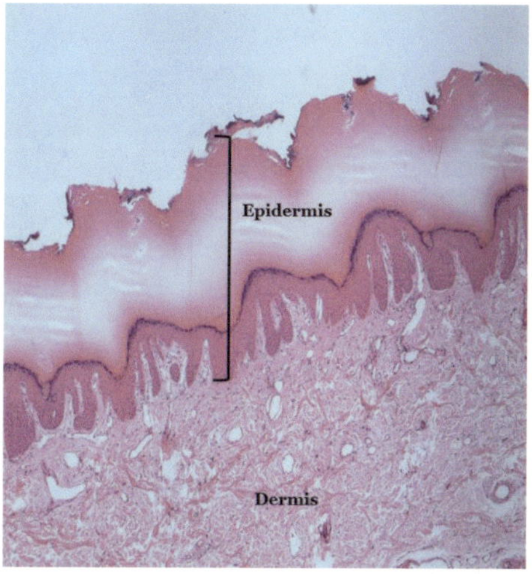

Figure 2.
Light microscopic image of the epidermis, skin. Keratinized stratified epithelium can be seen in the brackets. Hematoxylin–eosin staining (Dr. Alpaslan Gokcimen).

that forms the proximal and distal tubule, which allow the transport of the water and minerals. A rich capillary network exists around the basal invaginations. The cells pump the ions, glucose, sodium, potassium, and calcium through active transport from lumens of the tubes to the recesses. Thus, the water passes from the cytoplasm to the spaces that become hypertrophic and swell and expand, and then the collected water and ions pass into the veins [4, 9].

e. Avascularity: The epithelium is fed by diffusion through the blood vessels in the connective tissue below. In the feeding of multilamellar epithelium such as the skin, lip, esophagus, and vagina, the underlying connective tissue sends finger extensions into the epithelium. This is the name given to the "papilla" and thus feeding the epithelium [4, 5, 8].

f. Layer: The epithelial tissue can be classified according to the number of cell layers and the shape of cells. Different kinds/forms of epithelium are present in various organs, as shown in **Table 1**.

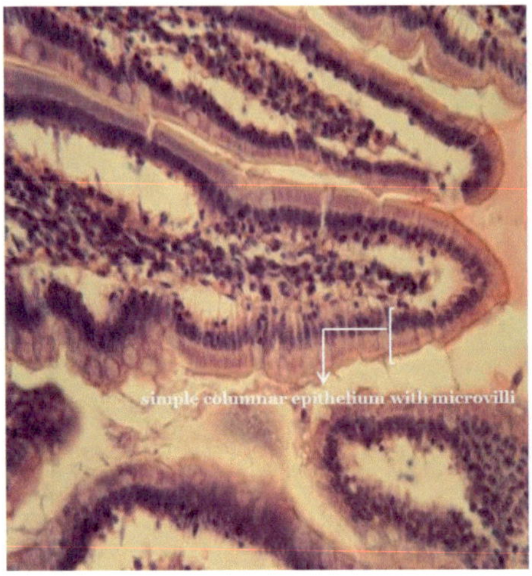

Figure 3.
Simple columnar epithelium with microvilli of the small intestine. Hematoxylin–eosin staining (Dr. Alpaslan Gokcimen).

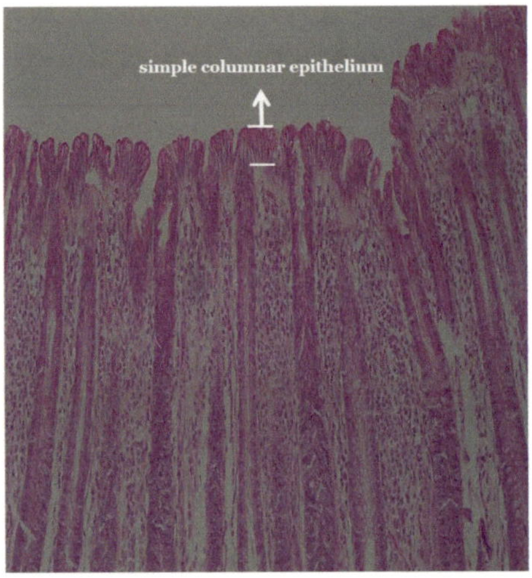

Figure 4.
Simple columnar epithelium of the large intestine can be seen between the lines. Hematoxylin–eosin staining (Dr. Alpaslan Gokcimen).

1.2 Functions of epithelial tissue

a. Protection against tearing and abrasion and protection against drying with keratin and mucus

b. Absorption of kidneys and intestines with microvilli

c. Surface transition: superficial transport with cell kinocilium

d. Secretion of hormones, digestive enzyme, and mucus

e. Sensory perception: taste buds, olfactory epithelium

f. Contraction: myoepithelial cells in glands [4, 6, 7, 10]

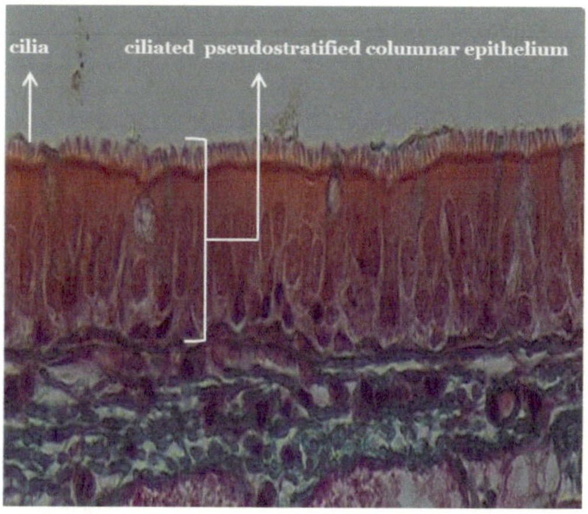

Figure 5.
Ciliated pseudostratified columnar epithelium of the trachea, Masson's trichrome staining (Dr. Alpaslan Gokcimen).

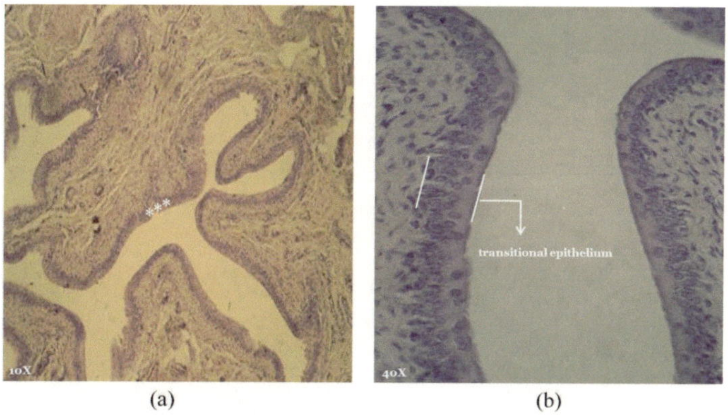

Figure 6.
(a) The transitional epithelium of the bladder. (b) The transitional epithelium of the bladder is marked at larger magnification Light microscopic image of bladder with transitional epithelium. Epithelium is shown by stars and between the lines. Hematoxylin–eosin staining (Dr. Alpaslan Gokcimen).

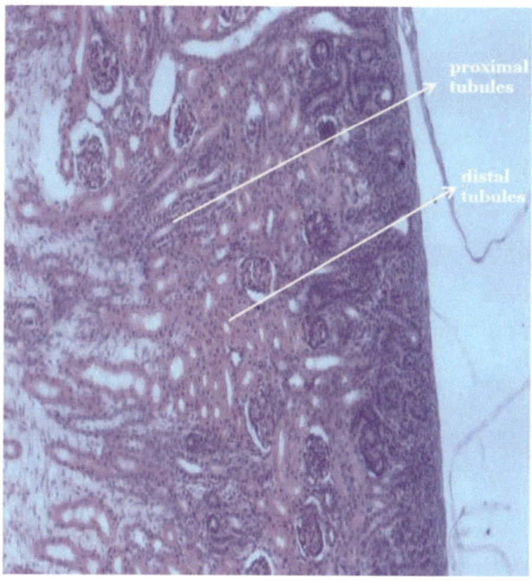

Figure 7.
Proximal and distal tubules of the kidney. Proximal tubules are the one which stained darker than the distal tubules. Hematoxylin–eosin staining (Dr. Alpaslan Gokcimen).

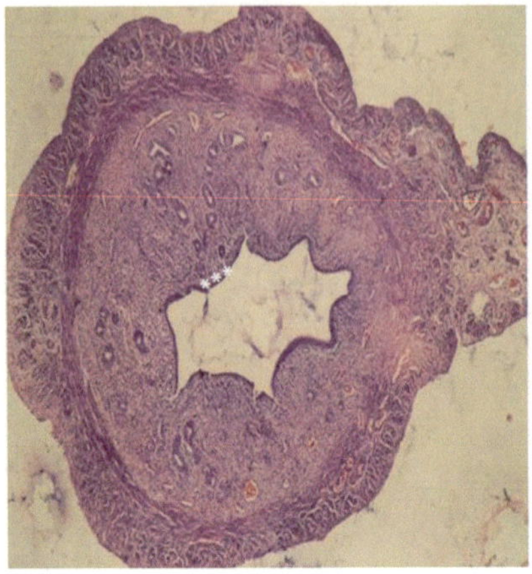

Figure 8.
Light microscopic image of the uterus with ciliated columnar epithelium. Epithelium is shown by stars. Hematoxylin–eosin staining (Dr. Alpaslan Gokcimen).

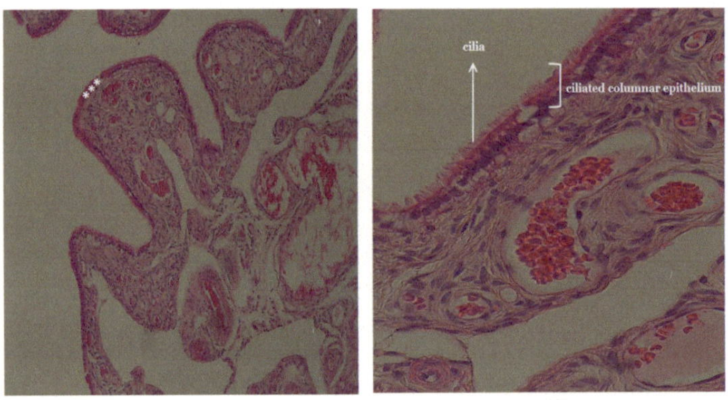

(a) (b)

Figure 9.
(a) Light microscopic image of the tuba uterina with ciliated columnar epithelium. (b) Epithelium is shown by stars and between the lines. Hematoxylin–eosin staining (Dr. Alpaslan Gokcimen).

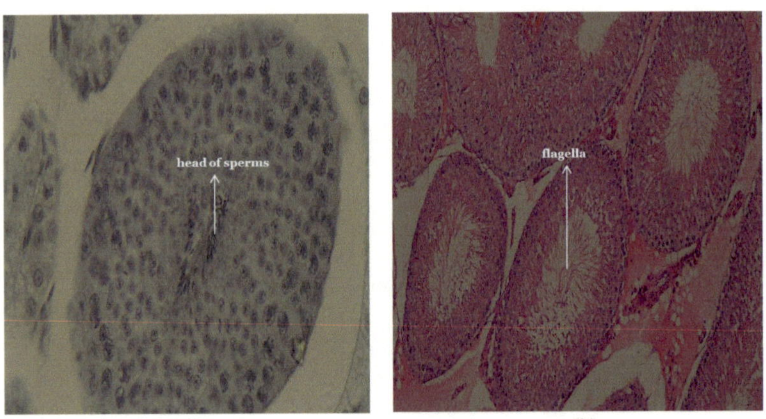

(a) (b)

Figure 10.
(a) Light microscopic image of seminiferous tubules, testis. Head of sperms and their flagellas can be seen. \(b) The figures show the iron hematoxylin–eosin staining, respectively (Dr. Alpaslan Gokcimen).

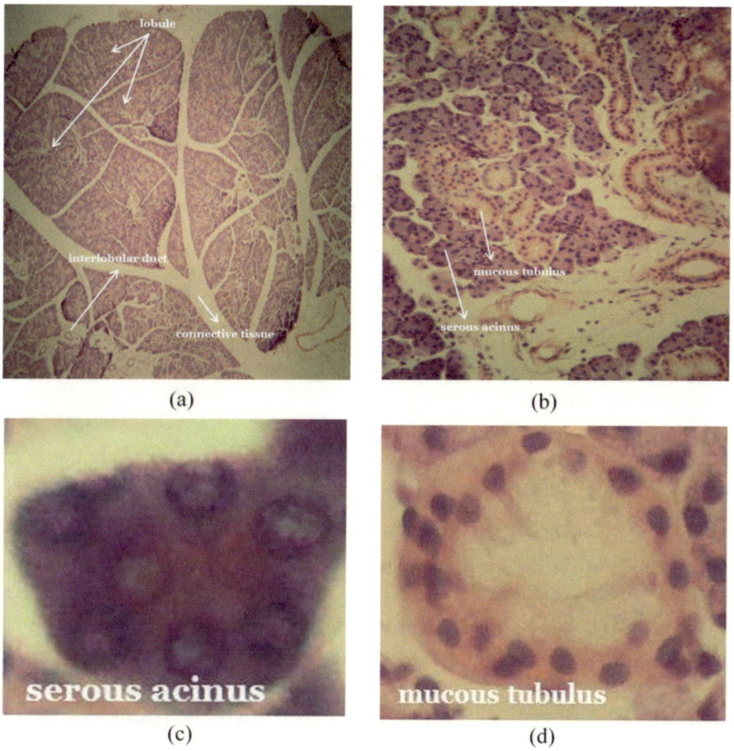

Figure 11.
(a) In the submandibular gland, irregular tight connective tissue is divided into lobules. Interlobular channels are seen in the connective tissue septa. (b) In the submandibular gland, serous acinus and mucous tubules are observed. Serous acini are predominant. (c) Serous acinus of the submandibular gland is observed. (d) The mucous tubule of the submandibular gland is seen (Dr. Alpaslan Gokcimen).

Type of epithelium	Places
Simple squamous epithelium	Parietal leaf of the kidney of Bowman capsule, serous membranes (peritoneum, pleura, mesothelium of the pericardium), vascular endothelium, type I alveolar epithelium laying lung alveoli.
Simple cuboidal epithelium	The proximal and distal of the kidney, the epithelium surrounding the colloid in the thyroid gland, the front face of the lens, the choroid plexus, the free face of the ovary, the most recent parts of the serous glands, the drainage channels of most glands and respiratory bronchioles. This type of epithelium allows the secretion and reabsorption of certain substances such as mucus, sweat, and enzyme.
Simple columnar epithelium	The stomach surface, small intestine and colon, gallbladder and uterine cavity.
Stratified squamous	This epithelium is divided into keratinized and non-keratinized. Keratinized epithelium is found in the skin and filiform papilla, non-keratinized epithelium is found in the lip, oral, pharynx, true vocal cords and vaginal epithelium.
Stratified cuboidal epithelium	Some sweat and salivary glands have this type of epithelium in the duct channels.
Stratified columnar epithelium	The female and male urethra, conjunctiva and large duct channels of some glands.
Transitional epithelium	In the urinary tract, from kidney and pelvis to a portion of the urethra. This epithelium is adapted to the short-term internal pressure

Table 1.
Types of epithelium and their locations [10].

1.3 Epithelium is classified as cover and secretory epithelium

1.3.1 Cover epithelium

The cover epithelium lines up the outer surface of the body and the inner surface of the hollow organs. The multilayer squamous epithelium, which forms the epidermis of the skin, has a protective effect by covering the outer surface of the body. Under the epithelium, there is a lamina propria and they are called as mucosa together and cover the inner surface of the cavities. Structures such as nasal mucosa, airway mucosa, digestive system mucosa, and urinary tract mucosa are good examples of laying lumen structures related to epithelial tissue [4–8].

1.3.2 Secretory epithelium

There are two types of glands—endocrine and exocrine.

a. The endocrine (hormone-producing) glands include the Langerhans islets of the pancreas, adrenal glands, and thyroid and parathyroid glands. Endocrine glands are supported by reticular fibers, arranged in cord or follicle. The most common cord shape is seen in the form of anastomoses around the capillaries or blood sinusoids. The produced hormone in the cell (adrenal gland, anterior lobe of the pituitary gland, parathyroid gland) is released through the appropriate signaling molecule or neural stimulus. In the follicular form of the endocrine gland, secretory cells surround the follicular cavity and store the produced hormone. The best example of this is the thyroid gland. Therefore, the endocrine glands do not have a discharge channel and deliver their secretions to the capillary network of the surrounding area [4].

b. Exocrine glands give their secretions to the external environment via a duct channel and are not rich in capillary network. Part of the pancreas, parotid, submandibular, and sublingual glands are the examples of exocrine glands [4–6, 8, 10].

There are irregular tight connective tissue sheath around the macroscopic glands which are parotid, submandibular, and sublingual gland. The connective tissue enters into the glands in the form of septa. The septa divide the gland into compartments. In the compartments, there may be acinus or tubules or both according to the type of the gland. Intralobulated duct channels are also included within the lobule. In the septa of connective tissue, interlobular channels are located. From these visible glands, the serous glands consist of acinus (alveolus), and the mucous glands are mucous tubules (**Figure 11a–d**). Exocrine glands can be subdivided into serous, mucous, and mixed glands according to the nature of the secretion they produce. Both serous- and mucous-secreting endpieces are covered with cubic epithelial cells which form intercalated (initial) ducts. Intercalated ducts combine to form the striated (intralobular) ducts. The intralobular ducts merge together to form the interlobular duct. These ducts are joined together and form "Stenson" in the parotid gland, "Wharton" in the submandibular gland, and "major sublingual" channels in the sublingual gland and open into the oral cavity. The most important features of intralobular ducts are the membrane folds extending from the cell basal to the nuclei. A large number of mitochondria were placed on the long axis of these folds. Such a location is particularly important for the salivary gland, which is functionally intense and consumes relatively more energy during its work. The parotid and the exocrine glands part of the pancreas are pure serous. The submandibular and sublingual glands are mixed glands [4–9].

1.3.3 Serous glands

The abundant zymogen granules in the serous glands are found in the upper part of the cell cytoplasm. Serous glands produce a smooth flow and protein secretion. The duct channels are narrower than the mucous glands. The nuclei of the cells are located in the middle and are round in shape. In the sections stained with hematoxylin–eosin, the basal part of the cell is stained with hematoxylin, and the apical portion is stained with eosin [4–8, 10] (**Figure 11c**).

1.3.4 Mucous glands

Mucous glands secrete carbohydrate properties. Since these granules are lost when preparing hematoxylin–eosin stained sections, these parts of the cells are often seen as empty. Therefore, these glands secrete in dense consistency and are lightly colored, and the discharge ducts are wider than the serous glands (**Figure 11d**) [4–9].

The epithelial cells of the gland are divided into three types according to the type of secretion:

1. Merocrine secretion: The secretory product is transported to the apical surface of the cell by vesicles. The vesicles are combined with the cell membrane and give their contents to the external environment by exocytosis. As in the pancreas, the most common form of secretion in the body is the merocrine type.

2. Apocrine secretion: While the secretory product is separated from the apical part of the cell membrane, it takes some cell membrane with it. This secretion occurs in the mammary glands, the apocrine of the skin, the ciliary (Moll's) of the eyelid, and the seromusin glands of the outer ear canal.

3. Holocrine secretion: Secretion product accumulates in the cell that continues to mature; then the secretory product is excreted into the outer environment together with the cell in which it is contained. The ovaries, the fat in the skin, and the Meibomian glands in the eyelid are the examples [4–8].

2. Structure of major salivary glands

a. The parotid gland is surrounded by irregular tight connective tissue called a capsule. The parts separated from the capsule move into the gland and are called septa. The septa separate the gland into lobules (**Figure 12a**). Each lobule is composed of spherical acini, which empty their serous secretion into intercalated ducts, from where it flows into striated (intralobular) ducts. We will see these ducts in the lobule. The intralobular ducts combine to form interlobular ducts. The interlobular ducts are located in the septa. Interlobular ducts leave the lobule and together with muscular arteries, veins, nerve, and lymphatic vessels. The interlobular duct channels are also known as excretory duct. Excretory ducts are emerged to form the main duct, "the Stenson." Round-shaped acinus is a part of the serous gland. The acinus (acinar cell) is formed by laying a single-layer cubic or prismatic epithelium on the basal lamina (**Figure 12b**). Fat cells which are one of the connective tissue cells are located between acini. Myoepithelial cells are located between epithelial cells and basal lamina. Contraction of myoepithelial cells accelerates the flow of saliva. Acinar secretion with serous content and secretion passes to intercalated ducts. Several intercalated ducts form an intralobular (striated) duct.

Prismatic-shaped epithelium is arranged on the basal lamina to form intralobular ducts. The basal cell membrane forms inward folds. A large number of mitochondria are located parallel to these basal invaginations. Basal invaginations are often seen in tissues and organs which allow water transport. The best example of this condition is the renal proximal and distal tubular epithelial cells and the striated duct in the salivary glands. Striated ducts have the ionic pump activity. These structures enable reabsorpsion of sodium and secretion of potassium and hydrogen ions, but reabsorption of sodium more than the potassium secretion. Thus, the secretion becomes hypotonic [7]. In this way, many substances which are reabsorbed from the apical are transported to the basal portion by active transport. The basal labyrinth is involved in transport of water and reabsorption of sodium from the saliva. Acinus and all excretory ducts are surrounded by a rich capillary network. The spherical-shaped nuclei of serous cells are in the middle of the cytoplasm. The organelles are well-developed granular endoplasmic reticulum and Golgi apparatus; the granular endoplasmic reticulum and ribosomes form ergastoplasm. Ergastoplasm is seen basophilic because it makes abundant protein synthesis. The ergastoplasm and Golgi complex together form secretory granules [4–10].

b. The submandibular gland as with the parotid gland has the irregular tight connective tissue that surrounds the organ and divides it into lobules (**Figure 11a**). The submandibular gland has both serous acinus and mucous tubules (the compound is a tubuloacinar gland), and the acinar cells were predominant. Hence, serous majority makes seromucous secretion. Acinus has the same structure as the parotid gland. The duct channels are also arranged in the same way as the parotid, and secretion is excreted in the oral cavity with "Wharton duct." The fat cells from connective tissue cells are located between the acinus and the mucous tubules. Myoepithelial cells are likewise located between the serous cells and the basement membrane and the basal membrane with mucous cells. A rich capillary system surrounds the organ. This system is accompanied by nerve vessels. Mucogenous granules are present in them because the mucous cells are pale. Since serous cells contain zymogen granules, they stained in dark color and have basophilic appearance. The ergastoplasm is dominant, and therefore, protein secretion is predominant to carbohydrate secretion [4–10].

c. The sublingual gland has the same structure as the other two major salivary glands. This gland is a mixed acinotubular. However mucous tubules are its predominant compound (**Figure 13a–d**). The duct channels of the gland, myoepithelial cells, and capillary and neural networks are as in the other two salivary glands, and salivary secretion reaches the oral cavity with a major sublingual duct. The fat cells are located between the functioning parenchyma [4–10].

d. The properties of macroscopic salivary glands are given in **Table 2**.

2.1 Structure of the lacrimal gland

The lacrimal gland is located on the upper lateral side of the orbit, beneath the conjunctiva (**Figure 14**). The lacrimal gland consists of several separate lobules formed by the tubuloacinar serous glands [7, 67]. The lacrimal gland is structurally similar to salivary glands. This gland was divided into lobules by irregular tight connective tissue. In the lobules, acinar cells and mucus tubules are located together. The acini have large lumens built with prismatic cells. Secretions produced in acinar and tubular structures are transmitted to the superior fornix

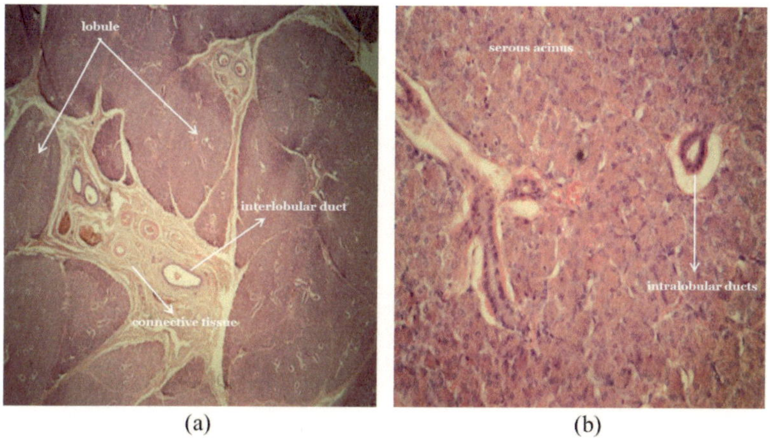

Figure 12.
(a) In the parotid gland, which is a pure serous gland, the irregular tight connective tissue is divided into the lobules. Interlobular ducts are seen. (b) Serous acinus and intralobular ducts are observed in the parotid section (Dr. Alpaslan Gokcimen).

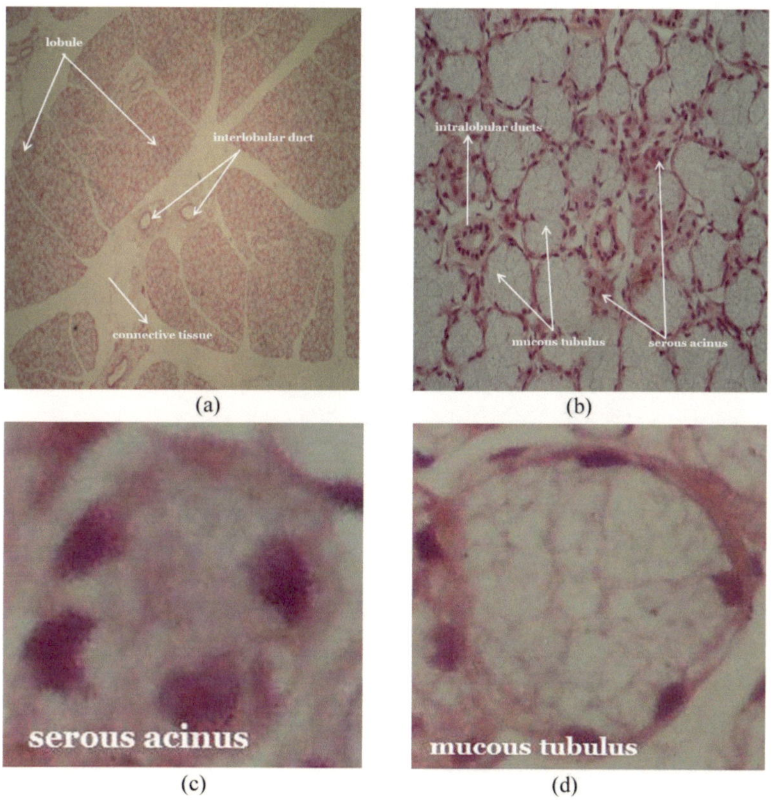

Figure 13.
(a) In the section stained with hematoxylin-eosin in the sublingual gland, the irregular tight connective tissue was divided into lobules. Interlobular ducts are observed. (b) The sublingual gland is a mixed gland consisting of mucous tubules and serous acini. Mucous tubules are predominant. (c) Serous acinus of the sublingual is observed. (d) The mucous tubule of the sublingual gland is seen (Dr. Alpaslan Gokcimen).

through the small duct channels. Tears drain in the inner aspect of the eye and then nasal cavity with the nasolacrimal duct (**Figures 15** and **16**), [10, 67]. The myo-epithelial cells located between the epithelial cells and the basal lamina help this process [4, 7].

Name of the gland	Secretory content	Structural properties of gland	The opening of the excretory channels into the mouth
Parotid Pure serous	Zymogen granules	Stroma: Irregular tight connective tissue Parenchyma: Asinus (Compound alveolar gland)	Intercalated channel Intralobular channel Interlobuler channel Excretory channel Stenon channel
Glandula submandibularis	Mainly serous mixed (serous and mucous) Zymogen and mucinogen granules	Stroma: Irregular tight connective tissue and ve fat cells Parenchyma: Compound tubuloalveolar gland	Intercalated channel Intralobular channel Interlobuler channel Excretory channel Wharton channel
Glandula sublingualis	Mainly mucous mixed (serous and mucous) Zymogen and mucinogen granules	Stroma: Irregular tight connective tissue and ve fat cells Parenchyma: Compound tubuloalveolar gland	Intercalated channel Intralobular channel Interlobuler channel Excretory channel Major sublingual channel

Table 2.
Comparison of secretory content, structure and discharge channels of saliva glands.

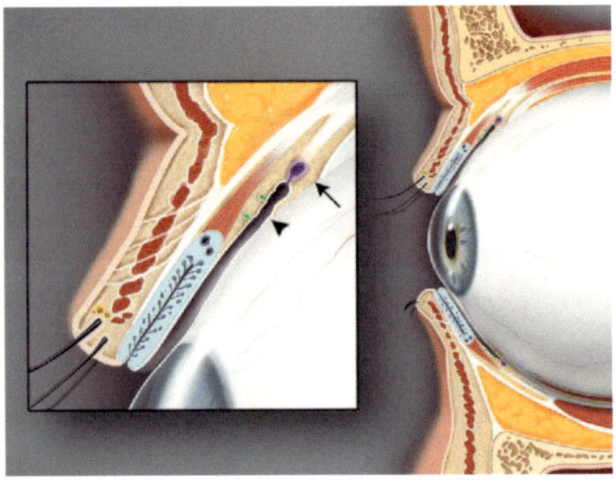

Figure 14.
Sagittal view of the upper and lower eyelids. The glands of Krause (arrow) are located in the superior conjunctival fornix. The glands of Wolfring (arrowhead) are found at the nonmarginal border of the tarsal plate [67] (with permission by Dr. Bhupendra Patel).

On the other hand, the lacrimal gland is made of several lobules separated by loose connective tissue. Each lobule consists of many acini, lined with columnar serous cells that produce a watery secretion. The central lumina of many units converge to form intralobular ducts, which unite to drain into 8–12 excretory ducts [11, 12].

2.2 The saliva and tear composition

Saliva is made up mostly of water (97–99.5%) originating from plasma of acinar cells [13]. The content of salivation has mucous, serous, or serous-mucous features. Mucous secretion is a thick form viscous fluid of highly glycosylated glycoproteins. Serous secretion is fluent and with clear consistency, forming thin, watery secretion containing proteins and glycoproteins. Seromucous form mixed secretin of intermediate thickness [14, 15]. Saliva is composed of a variety of electrolytes, including sodium, potassium, calcium, magnesium, bicarbonate, phosphates, immunoglobulins, proteins, enzymes, mucins, and nitrogenous products, such as urea and ammonia [16].

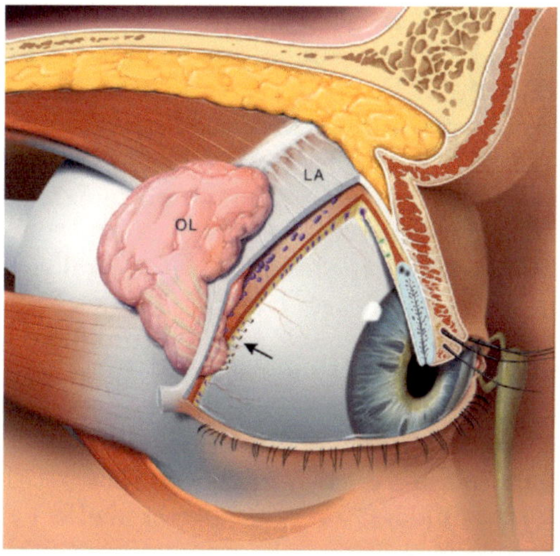

Figure 15.
Oblique view of the right orbit. Oblique view of the right orbit showing the main lacrimal gland divided into the orbital lobe (OL) and palpebral lobe by the lateral horn of the levator aponeurosis (LA). Note the excretory ducts coursing through the palpebral lobe and draining into the superior conjunctival fornix (arrow) [67] (with permission by Dr. Bhupendra Patel).

Histatins, the human salivary proline-rich proteins (PRPs) and statherin proteins are found in three kinds of protein saliva [17]. Histatins are a family of related neutral and basic histidine-rich peptides which are secreted mainly from parotid saliva and, to a lesser extent, submandibular saliva [18, 19]. A total of 12 salivary histatins have been isolated from human saliva.

The human salivary proline-rich proteins (PRPs) are a heterogeneous group of proteins that comprise about 70% of the parotid proteins. They are characterized by a predominance of the amino acids proline, glycine, and glutamic acid/glutamine (a total of 80% of all amino acids). PRPs are classified into three groups: acidic, basic, and glycosylated [20].

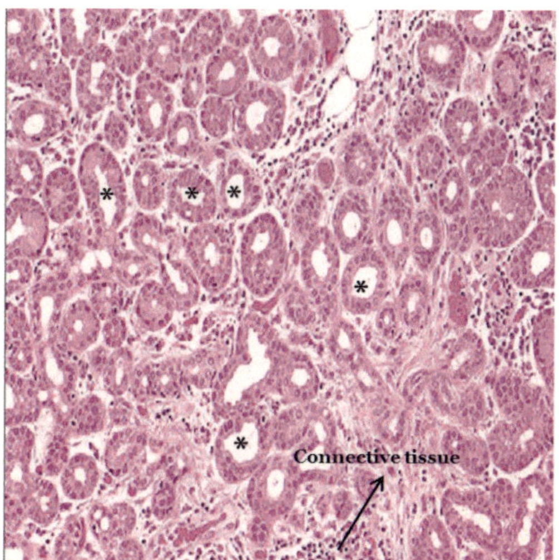

Figure 16.
Lacrimal gland histopathology. H&E staining of a normal lacrimal gland. The gland is composed of lobules separated by loose connective tissue. The lobules are composed of multiple acini lined by columnar secretory cells [67] (with permission by Dr. Bhupendra Patel).

Statherin is a low-molecular-weight acidic protein consisting of 43 amino acids. It is secreted by the parotid, submandibular, and von Ebner's salivary glands but is not present in labial saliva [21, 22].

Mucins are proteins that give the typical viscoelastic character to all the mucosal secretions (**Table 3**) [23–25].

Cystatins contain various kinds of endogenous proteinase inhibitors to regulate their protein metabolism or to protect tissues from proteolytic attacks by bacteria or viruses. Cystatins are important in the inhibition of several viruses, presumably by blocking necessary cysteine proteinases [26, 27].

Amylase is an abundant salivary component. It is produced mainly in the pancreas and salivary glands [17].

Secretory immune globulin A (slgA) is a member of the adaptive immune response [28, 29]. IgA, which is a connective tissue cell and located in the stroma, is secreted into the saliva by plasma cells [7, 30, 31].

Lysozyme is called muramidase, for its antibacterial effect also. It is a widely distributed enzyme occurring in many human secretions (**Table 3**).

Extra-parotid glycoprotein (EP-GP), an acidic salivary glycoprotein, was originally isolated from submandibular and sublingual saliva and has been shown to have a strong affinity to hydroxyapatite. EP-GP can be localized only in the serous acinar cells of the submandibular glands and is absent in the parotid gland [32].

Kallikreins are a group of serine proteases that are found in glandular cells, neutrophils, and biological fluids. Glandular (tissue) kallikrein is found in a variety of tissues and biological fluids, including saliva [33].

	Saliva	Tear fluid
Mucins	++++	+
Asidic PRPs	++++	–
α-Amylase	++++	+
Basic PRPs	+++	–
Basic PRG	+++	–
Secretory IgA	+++	++++
Cystatins	++	+
Statherin	++	+
IgG	+	+
EP-GP	+	+
VEGh	+	++++
Histatins	+	–
Lysozyme	+	++++
Kallikrein	+	
Lactoferrin	+	++++
Lactoperoxidase	+	+
Haptocorrin	+	+
β-Microseminoprotein	+	+
IgM	+	+
Albumin	+	+
Zn-α2 Glycoprotein	+	+

Table 3.
Comparison of saliva and tear secretion [17].

Haptocorrin is an acidic glycoprotein that is present as a minor component in blood and other body fluids. It binds cobalamin (vitamin B12) but should be distinguished from two other vitamin B12-binding proteins: the intrinsic factor and transcobalamin. In human salivary glands, haptocorrin has been localized only in mucous acinar cells and in intercalated duct cells where it can be released via β-adrenergic receptor stimulation [34].

β-Microseminoprotein is present in various amounts in mucous secretions [17].

Table 3 shows the distribution of saliva and tear content [17].

Tear fluid is a complex solution intended to sustain the surface of the eye [35]. The lacrimal gland secretes tear fluid consisted mainly of water and electrolytes, and human tears have been disclosed to be isotonic with plasma [36]. In the secretion of the lacrimal gland, lysozyme, which is the antibacterial enzyme, contains electrolytes close to the plasma concentration [10].

Lysozyme is mainly present in saliva and tear fluid, and it plays an important role in the protection of the oral cavity and eyes from infection.

In addition to salivary secretions, statherin is also present in tear fluid and nasal and bronchial mucus. Statherin prevents excessive precipitation of calcium salts in these fluids [17].

Haptocorrin at the highest concentrations have been detected in tears and nasal secretion [34].

2.3 Function of saliva secretion

Saliva is mainly secreted by the parotid gland, submandibular gland, and sublingual gland [16, 37, 38]. In addition, the mucosa of the mouth, the tongue, and the soft palate also contains large amounts of microscopic salivary glands and helps secretion.

Different substances and factors in saliva have various functions. These functions are listed below:

1. Digestion: Basically, saliva is composed of water (~99.5%); electrolytes such as potassium, sodium, bicarbonate, calcium, phosphorus, and chloride; and various enzymes, among other important elements. Enzymes include amylase, lipase, lysozyme, immunoglobulins, thiocyanate, and urea. Alpha-amylase enzyme breaks the glycosidic linkages of carbohydrates 1–4 and provides digestion of carbohydrates [7, 30, 31, 39].

2. Lubrication and protection: Since the intraoral food is the first fragmentation place, the sensitive and delicate oral mucosa should not be damaged. For this purpose, saliva secretion protects the oral mucosa, and saliva contains mucins, which allow it to coat and lubricate [31, 40, 41]. The most important feature of salivary secretion is that it lubricates and protects the very sensitive oral mucosa. The best lubricating components of saliva are mucins. Mucins also cause an antibacterial function by selectively modulating the adhesion of microorganisms to oral tissue surfaces [42, 43]. Chewing, speech, and swallowing all are provided by the lubricating effects of mucins [43]. Glycosylated basic PRPs (PRGs) function as masticatory lubricants and have also been shown to interact with several types of microorganisms such as *Fusobacterium nucleatum* [44]. The physiological functions of the mucins include cytoprotection, lubrication, protection against dehydration, and maintenance of viscoelasticity in secretions [44, 45]. The viscoelastic properties of mucins play a role in lubrication and are considered to be an important characteristic of mucins [25, 46]. The capacity of mucins to protect epithelial surfaces depends largely

on their high content of oligosaccharides and their ability to form a gel layer together with other salivary proteins [47]. Kallikreins have been implicated in the regulation of local blood flow in salivary glands [48].

3. Buffering action and clearance: Bicarbonates, phosphates, and urea act to modulate pH and the buffering capacity of saliva. Saliva plays an active role in the sense of taste. We get the sense of taste with "gemma gustativa" known as taste buds. With microvilli of these taste buds, it is possible to bathe with saliva secretion continuously and thus to recognize different tastes. The saliva also forms a medium for the suspended food materials so that the environment for the stimulation of the taste buds is formed [30, 40, 41]. The acini of serous glands first produce an isotonic fluid; and when the secretion product reaches the ductus striata, it is absorbed back into the sodium and secreted into the secretory potassium and bicarbonate, resulting in salivary isotonic-hypertonic; and due to the high concentration of bicarbonate ions, it buffers the contents of the oral cavity [7, 49]. Statherin, together with the acidic PRPs, plays a role in the calcium homeostasis of saliva [50, 51].

4. Mucins play a role in mucosal surface coating, creating a chemical barrier, as a component of saliva decides on its viscosity, and are a part of the immune system and are important in the adherence of the microbial flora [52].

5. Maintenance of tooth integrity: Calcium, phosphate, and proteins work together as an antisolubility factor and modulate demineralization and remineralization [16]. The acidic PRPs bind Ca^{++} with a strength that indicates that they are important in pellicle formation and in maintaining supersaturation of ionic calcium in relation to phosphate ions in saliva [53]. Therefore, the acidic PRPs may be of biological significance in maintaining the calcium homeostasis of saliva and in preventing the formation of salivary stones [54]. Acidic PRPs inhibit apatitic crystal growth, suggesting that, when adsorbed on the tooth surface, they block specific mineral growth sites [55]. Statherin bound to the enamel surface can inhibit crystal growth of hydroxyapatite [17]. Cystatins have been reported to bind to hydroxyapatite [17] and therefore may play a role in acquired pellicle formation. Cystatins have been shown to inhibit hydroxyapatite crystal growth [56].

6. Antibacterial activity: Immunoglobulins, proteins, and enzymes provide antibacterial action [16]. With intraoral secretion flow, the mucosa of the mouth remains moist, and also food residues and microorganisms are sent into the lumen of the digestive tract. Saliva makes this function with proteins and peptides that will neutralize all kinds of microorganisms. Therefore, in-house flora and hygiene are formed in this way [30, 40, 41]. Macromolecule proteins and mucins serve to cleanse, aggregate, and/or attach oral microorganisms and contribute to dental plaque metabolism. Especially in dental caries, systemic microorganisms are effective, and saliva secretion reduces the risk of systemic infection [30, 40, 41]. Histatins possess antimicrobial properties against a few strains of *Streptococcus mutans* [29] and inhibit hemagglutination of the periopathogen *Porphyromonas gingivalis* [57, 58] and neutralize the endotoxic lipopolysaccharides located in the outer membranes of Gram-negative bacteria, which may be an important part of the host's defense system [59]. Histatins are potent inhibitors of the growth and germination of *Candida albicans* [17]. Another biological role of histatins in the oral cavity is the inhibition of the release of histamine from mast cells, suggesting that they play a role in oral

inflammation [59]. The PRPs are thought to serve as a defense mechanism against dietary tannins by forming precipitates, which reduce harmful effects of tannins [60]. Statherin adsorbed onto hydroxyapatite can promote adherence of a few oral bacteria, such as *P. gingivalis* and *Actinomyces viscosus* [61]. Mucins promote the clearance of various bacteria by masking their surface adhesins, a factor which inhibits bacterial colonization [17, 62]. Salivary immunoglobulin A (slgA) associated response can be induced by local stimulation of mucosal membranes and secretory glands with antigens. Secretions of glands that are anatomically remote from the site of immunization, such as mammary, salivary, and lacrimal glands, can contain slgA antibodies to antigens encountered through the respiratory or gastrointestinal tracts. Following this pathway, IgA-producing cells are induced by the common mucosal immune response, consisting of lymphoid tissues concentrated in special structures, such as the Peyer's patches [17]. The protective role of slgA has been demonstrated in several experimental systems. Salivary immunoglobulin A can neutralize antigens (from viruses, toxins, and enzymes [63]. The enzymatic activity of lysozyme is able to cleave β-(1-4)-glycosidic bonds between muramic acid and N-acetylglucosamine residues in the peptidoglycan of the bacterial cell wall [64–66]. Haptocorrin play a role in the defense against microorganisms [17]. Beta-microseminoprotein has a protective function for the mucins by acting as a physiological inhibitor of endogenous mucin-degrading enzymes from leucocytes or by acting as an antibacterial agent [17].

7. Taste and digestion: Saliva plays an active role in the sense of taste. We get the sense of taste with "gemma gustativa" known as taste buds. With microvilli of these taste buds, it is possible to bathe with saliva secretion continuously and thus to recognize different tastes. The saliva also forms a medium for the suspended food materials so that the environment for the stimulation of the taste buds is formed [16, 30, 40, 41]. PRPs are involved in the bitter taste sensation [22].

2.4 Function of tear secretion

Tear secretion is extremely important for the health of the cornea and conjunctiva. Lacrimal secretions allow the creation of human tear film, made of the lipid, aqueous, and mucous layers. Tears, conjunctiva, and corneal epithelium are kept moist and remove foreign bodies. The tear film lubricates the surface of the eye, functions as a barrier against foreign body and microbial invasion, and supplies the avascular cornea with nutrients and oxygen [7, 67]. The tear covering the corneal surface in the form of a film layer is not homogeneous. Tear is mixture secretion and included the lacrimal glands, goblet cells, and eyelid tarsal gland secretions. The tear film layer includes proteins such as albumin and lactoferrin, enzymes such as lysozyme, lipids, metabolites, and electrolytes. The gland produces many proteins and aqueous fluid to add volume to the tear film. Furthermore, the lacrimal gland also secretes several bactericidal and fungicidal agents, akin to the salivary glands [11, 12]. Different isoforms of zinc α2-glycoprotein are present as a minor component in several body fluids, for example, serum, sweat, tears, and saliva [17].

"As a conclusion, the relation between the structure and function of exocrine glands is similar to other tissues. They produce normal secretions functionally as long as they maintain their normal shape and proper division of functions of individual cells. Saliva and tear secretion are necessary for survival, and these secretions are a barrier between environmental factors and internal organs. Tears and saliva are often the first line of defense, part of immune system, and element of transmission of information. These secretions constitute an important and even indispensable part of the body's functionality."

Author details

Alpaslan Gokcimen
Medicine Faculty, Department of Histology and Embryology, Aydın Adnan Menderes University, Turkey

*Address all correspondence to: agokcimen@yahoo.com

References

[1] Moore LK, Persaud TVN. The Developing Human. 6th ed. Philadslphia: W.B Saunders Company; 1988. 87 p

[2] Basaklar CA, editor. Medikal Embriyoloji. 11th ed. İstanbul: Palme Yayıncılık; 2011; 67, 74, 82 p

[3] Irez T, Erkan M, editors. Embriyoloji. 6th ed. İstanbul: Istanbul Tıp Kitapevi; 2016. 30 p

[4] Gokcimen A. Genel Tıbbi Histoloji. 11th ed. Isparta: Süleyman Demirel Üniversitesi Basımevi; 2006. 14, 30, 177 p

[5] Junqueira LC, Carneiro J. Basic Histology. 10th ed. Rio de Janerio: Lange International Edition; 2003. 170, 385, 369, 375, 376 p

[6] Paulsen FD. Histology and Cell Biology. 4th ed. Rio de Janerio: Lange International Edition; 2000. 58 p

[7] Baykal B. Histoloji Konu Anlatımı ve Atlas. 6th ed. İstanbul: Palme Yayıncılık; 2014. pp. 113-121

[8] Gartner PL, Hiatt LJ. Color Textbook of Histology. 2nd ed. Philadslphia: W.B Saunders Company; 2001. 91-95, 325, 332, 333, 339 p

[9] Kristic RV. Human Microscopic Anatomy. 3rd ed. Switzerland: Springer-Verlag; 1991. pp. 183-191

[10] Young B, Heath JW. Functional Histology. 4th ed. Toronto: Churchill Livingstone; 2000. pp. 81-85

[11] Garg A, Zhang X. Lacrimal gland development: From signaling interactions to regenerative medicine. Developmental Dynamics. 2017;**246**(12):970-980

[12] Yao Y, Zhang Y. The lacrimal gland: Development, wound repair and regeneration. Biotechnology Letters. 2017;**39**:939-949

[13] Ship JA, Fischer DJ. The relationship between dehydration and parotid salivary gland function in young and older healthy adults. Journal of Gerentology. 1997;**52**(5):310-319

[14] Finkbeiner WE, Shen BQ, Widdicombe JH. Chloride secretion and function of serous and mucous cells of human airway glands. The American Journal of Physiology. 1994;**267**(2 Pt 1): 206-210

[15] Salivary Glands and Saliva. VIVO Pathophysiology. 2017. Available from: http://pediaa.com/difference-between-serous-and-mucous/

[16] Humphrey SP, Williamson RT. A review of saliva: Normal composition, flow, and function. The Journal of Prosthetic Dentistry. 2001;**85**(2):62-169

[17] Schenkels LC, Veerman EC, Nieuw Amerongen AV. Biochemical composition of human saliva in relation to other mucosal fluids. Critical Reviews in Oral Biology and Medicine. 1995;**6**(2):161-165

[18] Oppenheim FG, Xu T, McMillan FM, et al. Histatins, a novel family of histidine-rich proteins in human parotid secretion. The Journal of Biological Chemistry. 1988;**263**(16):7472-7477

[19] Khurshid Z, Najeeb S, Mali M, et al. Histatin peptides: Pharmacological functions and their applications in dentistry. Saudi Pharmaceutical Journal. 2017;**25**(1):25-31

[20] Carlson DM. Salivary proline-rich proteins: Biochemistry, molecular biology, and regulation of expression. Critical Reviews in Oral Biology and Medicine. 1993;**4**(3/4):495-502

[21] Hay DI, Smith DJ, Schluckebier SK, et al. Relationship between concentration of human salivary

statherin and inhibition of calcium phosphate precipitation in stimulated human parotid saliva. Journal of Dental Research. 1984;**63**(6):857-863

[22] Azen EA, Hellekant G, Sabatini LM, et al. mRNAs for PRPs, statherin and histatins in Von Ebner's gland tissues. Journal of Dental Research. 1990;**69**(11):1724-1730

[23] Marxena E, Mosgaarda MD, Pedersenb AML, et al. Mucin dispersions as a model for the oromucosal mucus layer in in vitro and ex vivo buccal permeability studies of small molecules. European Journal of Pharmaceutics and Biopharmaceutics. 2017;**121**:121-128

[24] Löfgren D, Johansson D, Bohlin L, et al. The challenge of measuring viscoelastic properties of human whole saliva to fit clinical purpose. International Journal of Oral and Dental Health. 2015;**1**(4):1-6

[25] Van der Reijden WA, Veerman EC, Nieuw Amerongen AV. Shear rate dependent viscoelastic behavior of human glandular salivas. Biorheology. 1993;**30**(2):141-152

[26] Kopitar-Jerala N. The role of cysteine proteinases and their inhibitors in the host-pathogen cross talk. Current Protein and Peptide Science. 2012;**13**(8):767-775

[27] Bjorck L, Grubb A, Kjellen L. Cystatin C, a proteinase inhibitor, blocks replication of herpes simplex virus. Virology. 1990:941-943

[28] Mestecky I, McGhee JR. Immunoglobulin A (IgA): Molecular and cellular interactions involved in IgA biosynthesis and immune response. Advances in Immunology. 1987;**40**:153-245

[29] MacKay BJ, Denepitiya L, Iacona VJ, et al. Growth inhibitory and bactericidal of human parotid salivary histidine-rich polypeptides on Streptococcus mutans. Infection and Immunity. 1984;**44**(3):695-701

[30] Schipper RG, Silletti E, Vingerhoeds MH. Saliva as research material: Biochemical, physicochemical and practical aspects. Archives of Oral Biology. 2007;**52**(12):1114-1135

[31] Carpenter GH. The secretion, components, and properties of saliva. Annual Review of Food Science and Technology. 2013;**4**:267-276

[32] Veerman EC, van den Keybus PA, Vissink A, et al. Human glandular salivas: Their separate collection and analysis. European Journal of Oral Sciences. 1996;**104**(4Pt1):346-352

[33] Wong RS, Madapallimattam G, Bennick A. The role of glandular kallikrein in the formation of a salivary proline-rich protein A by cleavage of a single bond in salivary protein C. The Biochemical Journal. 1983;**211**(1): 35-44

[34] Nexø E, Hansen M, Olsen PS, et al. Salivary secretion of rat haptocorrin and amylase is stimulated by vasoactive intestinal polypeptide. Digestion. 1987;**36**(1):18-23

[35] Rolando M, Zierhut M. The ocular surface and tear film and their dysfunction in dry eye disease. Survey of Ophthalmology. 2001;**45 Suppl 2**: 203-210

[36] Tiffany JM. Tears in health and disease. Eye. 2003;**17**:923-926

[37] Young B, O'Dowd G, Woodford P. Wheater's functional histology. In: A Text and Colour Atlas. 6th ed. Toronto: Churchill Livingstone; 2013. pp. 184-464

[38] Farnaud SJ, Kosti O, Getting SJ, et al. Saliva: Physiology and

diagnostic potential in health and disease. Scientific World Journal. 2010;**10**:434-456

[39] Karn RC, Malacinski GM. The comparative biochemistry, physiology, and genetics of animal co-amylase. Advances in Comparative Physiology and Biochemistry. 1978;7:1-103

[40] Dawes C, Pedersen AM, Villa A, et al. The functions of human saliva: A review sponsored by the World workshop on oral medicine VI. Archives of Oral Biology. 2015;**60**:863-874

[41] de Almeida PV, Grégio AM, Machado MA, et al. Saliva composition and functions: A comprehensive review. The Journal of Contemporary Dental Practice. 2008;**9**:72-80

[42] Slomiany BL, Murty VL, Poitrowski J, et al. Salivary mucins in oral mucosal defense. General Pharmacology. 1996;**27**:761-771

[43] Tabak LA. Structure and function of human salivary mucins. Critical Reviews in Oral Biology and Medicine. 1990;**1**:229-234

[44] Gillece-Castro BL, Prakobphol A, Burlingame AL, et al. Structure and bacterial receptor activity of a human salivary proline-rich glycoprotein. Journal of Biological Chemistry. 1991;**266**:17358-17368

[45] Levine MJ, Reddy MS, Tabak LA, et al. Structural aspects of salivary glycoproteins. Journal of Dental Research. 1987;**66**:436-441

[46] Gans RF, Watson GE, Tabak LA. A new assessment in vitro of human salivary lubrication using a compliant substrate. Archives of Oral Biology. 1990;**35**:487-492

[47] Bradway SD, Bergey EJ, Scannapieco FA, et al. Formation of salivary mucosal pellicle: The role of transglutaminase. The Biochemical Journal. 1992;**284**:557-564

[48] Berg T, Carretero OA, Scicli AG, Tilley B, Stewart JW. Role of kinin in regulation of rat submandibular submandibular gland blood flow. Hypertension. 1989;**14**:73-80

[49] Kondo Y, Nakamoto T, Jaramillo Y, et al. Functional differences in the acinar cells of the murine major salivary glands. Journal of Dental Research. 2015;**94**(5):715-721

[50] Hay DI, Schluckebier SK, Moreno EC. Saturation of human salivary secretions with respect to calcite and inhibition of calcium carbonate precipitation by salivary constituents. Calcified Tissue International. 1986;**39**(3):151-160

[51] Raj PA, Johnsson M, Levine MI, Nancollas GH. Salivary statherin. The Journal of Biological Chemistry. 1992;**267**:5968-5976

[52] Ruhl S. The scientific exploration of saliva in the post-proteomic era: From database back to basic function. Expert Review of Proteomics. 2012;**9**(1):85-96

[53] Gibbons RJ, Hay DI. Human salivary acidic proline-rich proteins and statherin promote the attachment of Actinomyces viscosus LY7 to apatitic surfaces. Infection and Immunity. 1988;**56**(2):439-445

[54] Saitoh E, Isemura S, Sanada K. Inhibition of calcium- carbonate precipitation by human salivary proline-rich phosphoproteins. Archives of Oral Biology. 1985;**30**:641-643

[55] Aoba T, Moreno EC, Hay DI. Inhibition of apatite crystal growth by the amino-terminal segment of human salivary acidic proline-rich proteins. Calcified Tissue International. 1984;**36**(1):651-658

[56] Fujikawa H, Matsuyama K, Uchiyama A, et al. Influence of salivary macromolecules and fluoride on enamel lesion remineralization in vitro. Caries Research. 2008;**42**:37

[57] Gusman H, Travis J, Helmerhorst EJ, et al. Salivary histatin 5 is an inhibitor of both host and bacterial enzymes implicated in periodontal disease. Infection and Immunity. 2001;**69**(3):1402-1408

[58] Murakami Y, Tamagawa H, Shizukuishi S, et al. Biological role of an arginine residue present in histidine-rich peptide which inhibits hemagglutination of Porphyromonas gingivalis. FEMS Microbiology Letters. 1992;**98**:201-204

[59] Sugiyama K, Ogino T, Ogata K. Rapid purification and characterization of histatins (histidine-rich polypeptides) from human whole saliva. Archives of Oral Biology. 1990;**35**:415-419

[60] Mehansho H, Butler LG, Carlson DM. Dietary tannins and salivary proline-rich proteins: Interactions, induction and defense mechanisms. The Annual Review of Nutrition. 1987;7:423-440

[61] Kim SG, Hong JY, Shin SI, et al. Prevalence of *Porphyromonas gingivalis* fimA genotypes in the peri-implant sulcus of Koreans assessed using a new primer. Journal of Periodontal and Implant Science. 2016;**46**(1):35-45

[62] Toribara NW, Gum JR, Culhane PJ, et al. MUC-2 human small intestinal mucin gene structure-repeated arrays and polymorphism. Journal of Clinical Investigation. 1991;**88**:1005-1013

[63] Palomares O, Akdis M, Fontecha M, et al. Mechanisms of immune regulation in allergic diseases: The role of regulatory T and B cells. Immunological Reviews. 2017;**278**(1):219-236

[64] Goodman H, Pollock JJ, Katona LI, et al. Lysis of Streptococcus mutans by hen egg white lysozyme and inorganic sodium salts. Bacteriology. 1981;**146**:764-774

[65] Ito T, Yoshida Y, Shiota Y, et al. Effects of lectins on initial attachment of cariogenic Streptococcus mutans. Glycoconjugate Journal. 2018;**35**(1):41-51

[66] Lenander-Lumikari M, Loimaranta V. Saliva and Dental Caries. Advances in Dental Research. 2000;**14**:40-47

[67] Conrady CD, Joos ZP, Patel BC. Review: The lacrimal gland and its role in dry eye. Journal of Ophthalmology. 2016;**2016**:7542929. DOI: 10.1155/2016/7542929. [Epub 2016 Mar 2]

Chapter 3

Sjögren's Syndrome as an Ocular Problem: Signs and Symptoms, Diagnosis, Treatment

Dorota Kopacz and Piotr Maciejewicz

Abstract

Sjögren's syndrome (SS) is an autoimmune disease of exocrine glands, which is characterized by dry mouth and dry eye, though ocular disturbances, such as dry eye disease, may be the first sign of the problem. In pathogenesis of SS, activated T-cells and B-cells infiltrate the lacrimal glands and autoimmune process leading to cell destruction. This process causes hyposecretion of tears and aqueous-deficient dry eye disease. Evaporative dry eye disease is connected with Meibomian gland dysfunction (MGD) and/or goblet cell loss. There are many questionnaires and tests to dry eye disease diagnosing, but there is no "gold standard." Correlation of data from symptom questionnaires and results of ocular staining score, Schirmer test I (without anesthesia), and break-up-time make it easier to diagnose. The treatment of SS includes both local (tear drops and moistures) and systemic (nonsteroidal anti-inflammatory drugs—NSAIDs, glucocorticoids, and disease-modifying anti-rheumatic drugs—biologics) therapies, but it is individual. We would like to present recent data on the ocular involvement and perspective of dry eye disease diagnosis and treatment in patients with SS.

Keywords: dry eye, Sjögren's syndrome, pathogenesis, diagnostic tests and questionnaires, topical therapy, immunomodulatory therapy

1. Introduction

Sjögren's syndrome (SS) is a rheumatic autoimmune disease in which exocrine glands (salivary and lacrimal glands) are involved that results in clinical symptoms of dry mouth and dry eye. For the first time, SS-like clinical condition was described by Mikulicz in 1892 [1]. However, the disease was fully described (clinically and histopathology) later by the Swedish ophthalmologist Henrik Sjögren in 1930. He detected coincidence of rheumatism and hyposecretion of lacrimal and salivary glands and introduced the new term *keratoconjunctivitis sicca* to describe significant conjunctival and corneal staining with both dyes: methylene blue and rose bengal [1–3]. He also compared keratoconjunctivitis sicca and xerophthalmia seen in vitamin A deficiency and postulated that these cases represented a systemic disease. His doctoral thesis on this problem did not receive recognition and the author was disqualified from receiving PhD. Though his academic career was over, he lived on the day when the disease was named after him [2].

SS affects the exocrine glands; lymphocytic infiltration leads to sicca syndrome of the eyes, oral cavity, pharynx, larynx, and/or vagina [1, 3–6]. Systemic manifestations of SS are divided into visceral (lung, heart, kidney, endocrine, nervous system, gastrointestinal) and non-visceral (skin, myalgia, arthralgia). The risk of lymphoma is higher in patients with SS than in general population [1, 4, 6–8]. SS can be primary-pSS (without any other accompanying symptoms) or secondary-sSS (with other autoimmune diseases: systemic lupus erythematosus (SLE), rheumatoid arthritis (RA), polyarteritis nodosa, systemic sclerosis, granulomatosis with polyangiitis (GPA), primary biliary cholangitis (PBC), mixed connective tissue disease, occult thyroid eye disease) [1, 3–6, 9–11].

Dry eye disease (DED) problems are involved in diagnostic criteria of SS as an important part of diagnosis. Patients with DED seek medical help for many years prior to SS diagnosis—about 25% of DED patients have an underlying rheumatic condition, commonly pSS. Only one-third of patients with SS carried final diagnosis prior to ocular symptoms [1, 11, 12]. Some studies demonstrated coincidence of DED and SS in 46.7% cases [1, 11].

2. Pathophysiology

Primary Sjögren's syndrome is a multifactorial disorder including genetic predisposition, hormonal, and environmental factors [6, 13]. The pathogenesis of SS is incompletely understood. For years, it has been considered as T-cell dependent autoimmune response; now, the role of B cells is also described and is known as important. Tissue destruction is associated with the infiltration by both activated T and autoreactive B cells [1, 4, 6].

Plasmacytoid dendritic cells produce interferon (IFN)-I responsible for apoptosis/necrosis of glandular epithelial cells—it upregulates the major histocompatibility complex (MHC) molecules (class I and II) and costimulatory molecules (CD80,CD86), promotes production of cytokines (interleukin IL-6, IL-10, IL-12, IL-15, IF-γ, tissue growth factor TGF-β, tumor necrosis factor TNF-α), and chemokines (CXCL-11, CXCL-12, CXCL-13, CXCL-21) responsible for leukocytes migration resulting activation of the inflammatory reaction [1, 4, 6, 14, 15].

Glandular epithelial cells' necrosis/apoptosis reveals Sjögren-specific antibodies A (SSA, anti-RO) and B (SSB, anti-La)—though the role of these autoantigens is not completely clear, but the presence of them is one of the diagnostic criteria of pSS [1, 4]. Moreover, the presence of macrophage-derived chemokine (MDC) and thymus-activation-regulated chemokine (TARC), abnormal distribution of aquaporin (AQP)-5 cell membrane transporter, and defect in AQP-5 trafficking increased B-cell-activating factor (BAFF) and the matrix metalloproteinases (MMP) level were described in relationship with tissue damage in pSS [1, 4, 15–17].

Autoantibodies against type-3 muscarinic acetylcholine receptors are the suggested reason of peripheral neuropathies (PN) associated with SS though it has not been proved yet [6, 18].

3. Classification criteria

To standardize the diagnosis in patients taking part in clinical studies, to analyze results, and to facilitate the comparison of patients between centers, the classification criteria should be established.

In 1993, the Preliminary European Classification criteria for SS were published, and for almost 10 years have been the base for clinical, observational, and interventional studies [6, 19]. In 2002, the American-European Consensus Group (AECG) published a revised version of the SS classification criteria [6, 20–22]. All documents include ocular disturbances. AECG criteria for DED consist of symptoms and signs. Positive response to one question: (1) Have you had daily, persistent, troublesome dry eyes for >3 months? (2) Do you have a recurrent sensation of sand or gravel in the eyes? (3) Do you use tear substitutes >3 times a day? or positive one of tests: Schirmer without anesthesia ≤ 5 mm/5 min or vital dye staining of the ocular surface (≥4 van Bijsterveld or Ocular Staining Score OSS ≥ 5, [19–23]).

Because of their restrictive nature, the American College of Rheumatology approved the Sjögren's International Collaborative Clinical Alliance (SICCA) approach in 2012. To diagnose SS with ACR/SICCA criteria at least 2 of 3 are necessary: (1) a positive serum anti-Ro/-SSA or/and anti-La/SSB or [positive rheumatoid factor RF and antinuclear antibody (ANA) ≥ 1:320], (2) focal lymphocytic sialadenitis defined as focus score ≥ 1 focus/4 mm^2 in labial salivary gland biopsy samples, (3) OSS ≥ 3 [6, 21, 23].

Main differences between ACR/SICCA and AECG criteria are: (1) no subjective ocular and buccal symptoms and morphological or functional tests for salivary glands, (2) new OSS proposed by SICCA as the only test for ocular problems, (3) the association of RF positivity and ANA titer 1:320 as equivalent to anti-SSA/-SSB positivity [6, 21].

In 2016, ACR and EULAR published new pSS criteria containing again the Schirmer test and OSS in the dry eye assessment, as well as the test of unstimulated saliva production as a measuring tool for dryness in the mouth. The assessment of minor salivary gland biopsies and confirmation of the presence of the SS-A/Ro antibody were of particular importance. The remaining autoantibodies were not considered to be peculiar enough to diagnose pSS [21].

4. Ocular manifestation of SS

The main ocular manifestation of SS is DED. It is mainly a result of impaired lacrimal gland function due to inflammatory tissue damage. Hyposecretion of tears leads to aqueous-deficient DED. Moreover, exocrine glands of conjunctiva are also affected in SS and in connection with goblet cells reduction reveal evaporative DED [1, 6, 9, 22]. Ocular surface inflammation with conjunctival hyperemia and corneal epithelial damage leads to functional vision impairment [1, 2, 6, 22, 24]. Squamous metaplasia of the ocular surface epithelium, follicular conjunctivitis, corneal epitheliopathy, filamentary keratitis, sterile infiltrates, scleritis, poor epithelial integrity, recurrent erosions, dysesthesia, corneal ulceration, vascularization, opacification, and sometimes perforation were also described in SS patients [1, 2, 6, 22, 25].

5. Diagnostic procedures for DED

Dry eye disease among other diseases is the symptom causing the greatest morbidity and impairment of quality of life. Therefore, the patient is actively seeking a medical help. DED is typically diagnosed by evaluation of both eye symptoms and results of eye examination that symptoms not always match signs. Some patients have no symptoms though they have changes of ocular surface and others have significant eye discomfort, but there are very little signs in eye examination [1, 2, 22, 26–28].

5.1 Symptoms

Three characteristics features define DED: symptoms of discomfort, visual disturbance, and tear film instability with potential damage of ocular surface [9, 22, 28]. The discomfort is described as itching, stinging, burning, "foreign body sensation," or, occasionally pain. Visual disturbance means fluctuation of vision, especially during reading or working at a computer. In those cases, blinking recovers the vision [22, 28].

There are several questionnaires for the assessment of DED symptoms: Ocular Surface Disease Index (OSDI), the McMonnies questionnaire, the Impact of Dry Eye on Everyday Life survey (IDEEL), the Symptom Assessment in Dry Eye survey (SANDE), and the Standard Patient Evaluation of Eye Dryness questionnaire (SPEED). They are used as screening tests for DED, to diagnose DED, to monitor changes over time, and to control effect of the therapy in both clinical practice and research [6, 22, 23, 28]. Schaumberg et al. proposed a short questionnaire for clinical DED screening. It consists of only three questions: (1) Have you ever been diagnosed by a clinician as having dry eye syndrome? (2) How often do your eyes feel dry/not wet enough? and (3) How often do your eyes feel irritated? [28–30]. It has turned out that 2 specific symptoms quarried (dryness and irritation) are equivalent to asking up to 16 symptom questions [28, 31].

5.2 Signs

Evaluation of DED considers on: tear function, tear composition, and ocular surface changes.

The biomicroscopic examination evaluates luster and integrity of the tear film, the marginal tear strip, debris, and inflammatory cells in the tear film. The marginal tear strip is normally 1 mm in height and in DED is reduced. In clinical practice, a tear meniscus below 0.2 mm is regarded as pathological [2, 6, 9, 22, 25, 28, 32]. It is observed with the wide beam of the light and measured with narrow beam or optical instruments (description of those instruments and the interpretation of their measurements are available on the Tear Film and Ocular Surface Society website; www.tearfilm.org) [9, 28]. Corneal filaments are responsible for uncomfortable or painful sensation of patients [28] **Figure 1—(1)**.

Tear film instability is produced by either aqueous-deficient or evaporative or a combination of both mechanisms of DED. It can be also effect of ocular surface irregularities. To determine tear film stability tear film break-up time (TBUT) is used. The fluorescein dye is placed into the tear film and slit lamp with cobalt blue filtered light examination is performed: breakup is determined by a dark spot forming in the tear film. Normal BUT is greater than 10 s [2, 6, 9, 22, 28]. Devices using computer-analyzed reflections from the cornea has also been used for noninvasive tear stability analysis (noninvasive tear film break-up time NITBUT) [9, 28, 32–34] **Figure 1—(3)**.

The Schirmer test is described as "test to measure change in tear volume (production)" [9, 22]. A small strip of filter paper (5 × 35 mm) is placed on the margin of lower eyelid at the junction of the lateral and middle third of the lid. After 5 min, wetting of the strip is measured. If the test is performed without anesthesia-reflex tearing (e.g., tearing in response to a stimulus), the cutoff value is 5 mm; if the test is done after topical anesthesia-nonreflex (basal tears), the cutoff value is 3 mm [2, 6, 9, 22, 25, 28]. Although inter- and intraindividual differences were described, the range and absolute values are reduced in aqueous-deficient dry eye [7, 32]. Some clinicians use the phenol red thread test to measure tear volume; a small thread impregnated with phenol red dye is placed on the lower lid margin for 15 s. The normal value of the threat wetting is over 10 mm [9, 28, 32], **Figure 1—(2)**.

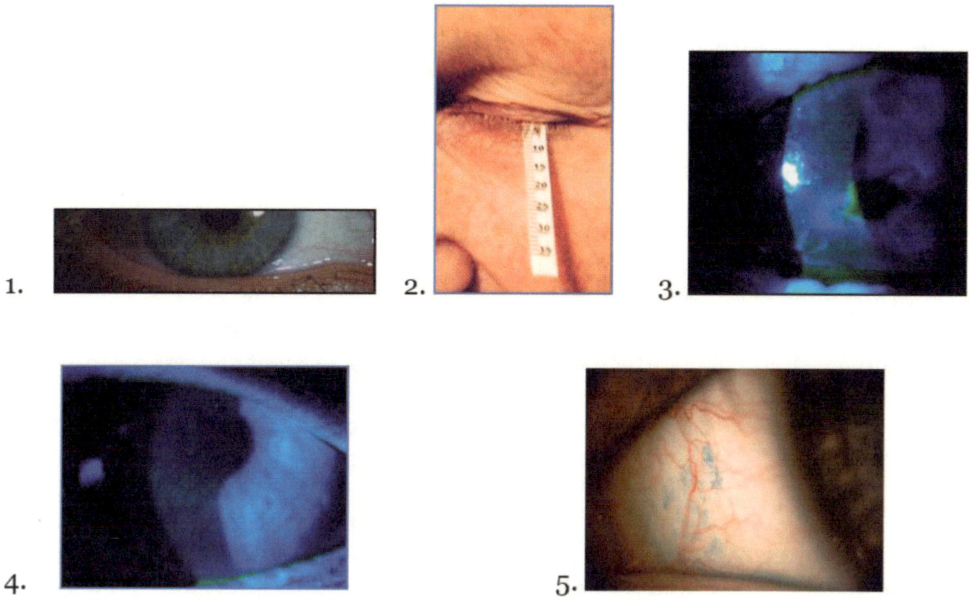

Figure 1.
Common diagnostic tests for dry eye disease: (1) tear film meniscus; (2) Schirmer test; (3) fluorescein break-up time; (4) fluorescein staining; and (5) lissamine green staining.

The tear film composition analysis includes measurements of tear osmolarity (TO) and levels of inflammatory mediators. Elevated osmolarity of the tear film is a characteristic for DED though there is no suggested cutoff value for SS-related DED and further investigations should be conducted to establish it [9, 28, 32, 35, 36]. There is positive correlation between TO and OSDI score and OSS and negative correlation between osmolarity and Schirmer I test [28, 37]. Some studies found that a higher TO was associated with lower OSDI score in SS patients that was connected with the less corneal sensitivity [35, 38, 39]. TO measurements of both eyes are recommended: in early stages of DED, transient lower TO was noted; the effect was asymmetrical and this effect was not seen in subject without DED [28].

Measurements of inflammatory mediators in the tear film help to identify the inflammatory reaction and the severity of DED [22, 28, 38]. The levels of various cytokines (TNF-α, IL-1α, IL-1ß, IL-6, IL-8, IL-10, IL-12P70, IL-13, MIP-1α, IFN-γ) and MMP-9 in tears of DED patients are significantly higher than those in normal people [22, 28, 40, 41]. Statistical differences among subclasses of DED for IL-8 and TNF-α were observed and it could be significant for diagnosing and treatment of DED [40]. The activity of cathepsin S (CTSS) in tears and the level of HLA-Dr in impression cytology were higher in patients with SS than in patients with non-SS DED and healthy subjects [22].

Ocular surface evaluation is commonly clinically performed with the instillation of topical dyes. Fluorescein and lissamine green (or rose bengal) are vital dyes used to determine the integrity of the cornea and conjunctiva. Fluorescein is used for corneal examination (it stains punctate erosions), lissamine green (or rose Bengal) for conjunctival staining (both dyes stain mucus strands, filaments, and areas of epithelium unprotected by normal glycocalyx) [2, 6, 9, 22, 28]. Staining indicates corneal surface disease: greater staining means greater severity of DED. Conjunctival staining usually occurs before corneal staining, medial before temporal conjunctival staining [9, 28]. To evaluate and grade staining there are several systems such as 1995 NEI/industry Workshop System, the Oxford System, the van Bijsterveld system, the Ocular Staining Score (OSS) developed by SICCA [9, 22, 25, 28, 32] **Figure 1—(4, 5)**.

Meibomian gland dysfunction (MGD) is defined as: "a chronic, diffuse abnormality of the Meibomian glands, commonly characterized by terminal duct obstruction and/or qualitative/quantitative changes in the glandular secretion; this may result in alteration of the tear film, symptoms of eye irritation, clinically apparent inflammation, and ocular surface disease" [22, 41, 42]. MGD is the common cause of evaporative DED. Studies of SS patients found that MGD is common problem of them; they have higher Meibomian gland dropout scores compared with healthy group and worse Meibomian gland expressibility compared to non-SS DED patients [22, 24, 43]. The lipid layer is an important factor for ocular surface health and tear film stability [22, 44]. The thickness of this layer (lipid layer thickness LLT) is changed in DED and MGD; healthy subjects have LLT thinner than DED [22, 24, 45–47].

Imaging of the ocular surface is a valuable tool to document and determine changes, as well as differentiate aqueous-deficient and evaporative DED. New devices perform minimally invasive objective measurements (no drops, no touching of the eye) of NITBUT, TMH, images of the Meibomian glands (meibography), bulbar redness, and LLT [9, 22, 47–50].

An in vivo confocal study demonstrated morphologic changes in corneas of SS patients: a decrease in central corneal thickness was hypothesized to be due to inflammatory process, a reduced number of subbasal plexus fibers may explain the phenomenon of decreased corneal sensitivity [51, 52].

6. Treatment of SS-related DED

Dry eye from SS is more severe than idiopathic one, so effective in idiopathic DED treatment may or may not work in SS. After diagnosing SS, the aim of the treatment is to maintain the tear film integrity through preservation, augmentation, and/or replacement of the deficient tear secretion [28, 51, 52]. There are many different therapies for DED, but there is no one treatment that works for everybody [22, 28, 32, 53, 54]. Though management approach of DED has changed over the years, some principles persist [28, 32, 54]. The treatment strategy is based upon the severity of DED and patients response to each added therapy. It includes patients' education, tears supplementation, management of MGD, inflammation of the ocular surface, and/or associated systemic disease [28, 32, 54].

6.1 Patient education

Good cooperation of the DED patient requires understanding by them the disease (chronic), the aggravating factors (e.g., cigarette smoke, dry heating air, air conditioning, low humidity, pollutions, systemic medications that reduce tear secretion), and the management strategy (long-term and possibly slow to take effect). Some modifications of environment and activities of daily living can improve patients' quality of life [28, 32, 54, 55].

6.2 Tear supplementation: artificial tears

Artificial tears are a standard of therapy for all severity grades of DED. The aim of this therapy in SS is to add tear film volume, to increase time of tear supplement on ocular surface and to reduce friction between lid and globe [28].

These preparations are not similar to natural tears: the main ingredients of them are lubricants or viscosity agents. Tear supplements varied in formulas: some of them include electrolytes, which are in normal tears to prevent ocular surface damage, some of them are hypotonic or distribute between the tear film and intracellular fluid to protect against the pro-inflammatory effect of tears hyperosmolarity. They are based on polyvinyl alcohol, povidone, hydroxypropyl guar, cellulose derivatives, and hyaluronic acid. To mimic lipid component of tears triglycerides, phospholipids, and castor oil are used. Depending on viscosity of the lubricant (macromolecular complexes that increase the residence time of the supplement in the tear film) and thickness of supplement they may cause blurred vision; gels are more viscous than solutions, ophthalmic ointments are the thickest of lubrications. Typically, ointments are used before bedtime to provide DED symptoms, enabling sleep [28, 32, 54, 56, 57].

Preservatives (benzalkonium chloride or EDTA) in the tear supplements are potentially toxic to the ocular surface (epitheliotoxic). The toxicity of them increases in patients with DED because of frequent use of drops and decreased tears volume. The usage of artificial tears more than 4–6 times a day requires preservative-free unit dose vials [28, 54, 58].

There is wide variety of tear supplements but none is clearly superior. "The main variables in the formulation of ocular lubricants regard the concentration of and choice of electrolytes, the osmolarity and the type of viscosity/polymeric system, the presence or absence of preservative, and, if present, the type of preservative" [28, 54].

Long-acting ocular surface lubrication is also achievable through the hydroxypropyl cellulose insert usage. The insert is placed in the inferior conjunctival fornix and dissolves at body temperature. Thickening the tear film it decreases the need for frequent topical lubrication, used at bedtime it substitutes the ointment [28, 54, 59].

6.3 Anti-inflammatory therapy

Since inflammation plays a key role in the pathogenesis of DED, many anti-inflammatory therapies have been evaluated in clinical trials and animal models. Better control of inflammatory reaction means DED symptoms and signs improvement.

6.3.1 *Topical corticosteroids*

There are some studies on short-term topical use of steroids in patients with SS and DED [9, 22, 28, 54, 60]. A 2- to 4-week course of treatment in patients with moderate to severe DED showed an improvement in both symptoms and signs: decreased symptom score, conjunctival hyperemia and corneal fluorescein staining, better TFBUT and Schirmer test measurements, higher numbers of goblet cells on impression cytology and lower numbers of inflammatory cells [28, 52, 60–63]. Topical steroids as a pulse therapy was noted as safe and effective one [60]. There are possible complications associated with long-term steroids usage: cataract, glaucoma, and infections. Elevated intraocular pressure and posterior subcapsular cataracts were described in patients using steroids over 3 months [28, 64].

6.3.2 *Topical cyclosporine A*

Cyclosporine A (CsA) is one of the powerful anti-T-cell immunosuppressive agents, but with no bone marrow suppression. The mechanism of action includes both inhibition of T-lymphocyte activation and other inhibitory properties, as the ability to inhibit apoptosis of other cells [28, 54, 65, 66]. Topical CsA reduce the cell-mediated inflammatory reactions [66] that results in improvement in symptoms (blurred vision, ocular dryness, foreign body sensation, and epiphora), reduction of fluorescein staining, better tear production (Schirmer test), reduction of pro-inflammatory cytokine and HLA-DR expression, increase of goblet cell density [2, 22, 28, 32, 67, 68]. Better tears production is probably connected with local release of parasympathetic neurotransmitters [32, 69]. CsA instilled to the conjunctival sac seems to be the first therapeutic (not only symptomatic as others) treatment for patients with moderate to severe DED due to aqueous deficiency [66, 70].

The use of topical CsA for evaporative DED due to MGD is recommended by the International Tear Film and Ocular Surface Workshop on Meibomian Gland Dysfunction [28, 54, 71]. Traditional treatment of posterior blepharitis and MGD include lid hygiene, massages, hot compresses, low-dose tetracyclines, and topical antibiotics [28, 32, 71]. In some studies, the CsA-treated patients had a greater decrease in the number of obstructed Meibomian gland, improvement in the viscosity of Meibomian gland secretion, TFBUT, staining scores, and Schirmer scores than those treated in traditional way [28, 72, 73].

Long-term study confirmed safety of topical cyclosporine in 3-year follow-up [28, 74].

6.3.3 Topical lifitegrast

Lifitegrast is a direct competitive antagonist of binding of lymphocyte function-associated antigen 1 (LFA-1) to intracellular adhesion molecule 1 (ICAM-1). Interaction between LFA-1 and ICAM-1 leads to T-lymphocyte adhesion to endothelial cells, migration to tissue, antigen presentation and recognition facilitating the formation of an immunological synapse. It releases inflammatory mediators, cytokines, chemokines, TNF-α, and IL-1 which are responsible for perpetuation and intensification DED inflammation [2, 22, 75–79]. The clinical efficacy of lifitegrast in patients with DED has been reported: improvement in symptom scores and ocular staining score in patients using it for 12 weeks. No serious ocular adverse events occurred [22, 75–79]. However, there are no studies comparing lifitegrast and other anti-inflammatory agents, evaluating whether lifitegrast in combination therapy could work better in DED—those problems need further studies [79].

6.4 Biological tear substitutes

6.4.1 Autologous serum

Serum is the fluid component of full blood that remains after clotting [54]. Human serum is similar to natural tears and contains many important components as: (1) epithelial growth factor EGF (acceleration of epithelial cell migration and anti-apoptotic effects); (2) transforming growth factor-ß/TGF-ß (involved in the epithelial and stromal repair process); (3) vitamin A (prevent epithelial squamous metaplasia and modulate the expression of thrombospondin-1); (4) thrombospondin-2, vascular endothelial growth factor A/VEGF-A, metallopeptidase-9 which with TGF-ß promote wound healing; (5) albumin (anti-apoptotic activity); (6) α-2 macroglobulin (exhibits anti-collagenase activity); (7) fibronectin (involved in cell migration); (8) substance P and insulin-like growth factor (potential role in corneal epithelial migration and adhesion); and (9) immunoglobulins and lysozyme (bactericidal and bacteriostatic effect). Significant improvement in symptoms, fluorescein TFBUT, and ocular surface staining score were reported after autologous serum drops treatment [28, 54, 80–82]. However, some studies reported no significant advantage in tear film stability, Schirmer test, or fluorescein staining in the use of AS over AF [83–85]. It is free of preservatives and has osmolarity and biomechanical properties similar to natural tears [54, 80, 84].

6.4.2 Autologous plasma

Plasma rich in growth factors (PRGF) and platelet-rich plasma (PRP) have been reported as successful treatment in DED patients [54, 84, 85]. Both of them (PRGF and PRP) are liberated from the platelets during preparation. Those components help in the proliferation, migration, and differentiation of corneal epithelial cells [84–87]. Both PRGF and PRP are preservative-free, well tolerated with almost no side effects [84–87]. Further investigations to compare them with other hemoderivatives and with commercial artificial tear eye drops are necessary.

6.5 Tear stimulation: secretagogues

"A secretagogue is a substance that causes another substance to be secreted" [28, 54]. Oral pilocarpine and cevimeline are indicated for treatment of dryness in SS. As muscarinic agonists, they stimulate secretion of saliva, aqueous tear from lacrimal glands, conjunctival epithelium, and mucin from goblet cells [52]. Some studies have shown their effectiveness in DED treatment in SS patients. The oral 10–30 mg/day of pilocarpine improves DED symptoms in comparison to placebo or artificial tears as well as a punctal occlusion. While there was no improvement in Schirmer test result, the patients with oral pilocarpine showed better score of ocular staining. Moreover, in SS patients with oral pilocarpine treatment increased the number of conjunctival goblet cells [28, 54, 88, 89]. The oral cevimeline dosage of 20–30 mg every 8 h improved ocular staining scores and TFBUT but no significant differences in lacrimal flow rates were found [28, 54, 90].

Topical secretagogues are approved in treatment of dryness in Japan. Drugs as: 2% rebamipide which increases mucin level over the conjunctiva and cornea (improves TFBUT), 3% diquafosol tetrasodium which increases mucin and fluid secretion (improves ocular staining) are introduced for DED topical treatment in clinical practice [22, 54, 91].

6.6 Tear retention

6.6.1 Punctal occlusion

The idea of punctal/canalicular occlusion is to block tear drainage from the ocular surface and use patients' own tears to maintain the lubrication of the eye. It also helps maintain instilled artificial tears longer [28, 54, 91]. The concept of permanent cautery lacrimal puncta occlusion for DED treatment was described in 1936, first dissolvable implants were used in 1961, but the modern idea of punctal plug use began with Freeman report in 1975 [54, 91–93]. Plugs are made of variety of materials and design, they can be absorbable (last 3 days to 6 months) or non-absorbable. The ideal occluder should be easy to place, block the drainage effectively, be biocompatible, long lasting, easy reversible, and have low potential for infection [28, 54, 91]. Punctal/canalicular plugs are common second-line treatment in aqua-deficiency DED. A comparison of plugs versus artificial tears in patients with SS and DED demonstrated that both treatments improved symptom scores, corneal staining and TFBUT, but Schirmer test and TFBUT were statistically more improved in plugs' group [28, 94].

6.6.2 Contact lenses

Therapeutic contact lenses (TCL) are used to promote corneal healing, protect the ocular surface from the lids and environment, reduce desiccation, and relieve discomfort [22, 28, 54]. Silicone-hydrogel materials have higher oxygen transmission than hydrogels. Some of soft silicone-hydrogel contact lenses are approved for therapeutic wear and could be useful in primary and secondary Sjögren syndrome for relief from discomfort and blurred vision. There is no literature on the use TCL in the treatment of DED in SS, but reports on such a treatment in other entities or ocular surface problems are encouraging [28, 52, 54, 95].

Bandage contact lenses (BCL) are large-diameter, rigid, gas-permeable lenses with scleral fixation. Retention of a fluid reservoir over the cornea and no corneal touch are the reason of the therapeutic effect of BCL. The use of BCL specifically in SS patients is not described, but some patients with SS were included in the groups in which benefit were demonstrated [28, 52, 54, 96].

6.7 Mucolytic therapy

Severe symptoms of eye surface irritation in patients with mucus filaments/strands are the reason to use topical mucolytic solution. Topical N-acetylcysteine (10–20% aqueous solution) therapy for 2–4 weeks usually resolves the problem [28, 97].

6.8 Essential fatty acids

Essential fatty acids (EFA) are polyunsaturated fats that are not synthesized by humans. Dietary supplementation (e.g., fish oil or flax seed oil or nutritional supplements) with omega-3 EFA as anti-inflammatory therapy is considered. Improvement in DED symptoms and signs with both oral and topical omega-3 EFA was described although there is nothing specific regarding the use for SS [22, 28, 97–8]. Gamma-linolenic acid is an omega-6 EFA with anti-inflammatory effect in chronic inflammatory diseases. An inverse association between it and levels of anti-SSA/anti-Ro antibodies were described. Improvement of symptoms and corneal staining after oral supplementation with omega-6 EFA were found [52, 99, 100].

6.9 Management of eyelids

MGD treatment include eyelid hygiene, hot compresses, eyelid massages, thermal pulsation treatment, anti-inflammatory, and antibacterial therapy (e.g., oral tetracyclines and EFA omega-3, topical azithromycin and EFA omega-3 [22, 28, 54, 71, 97, 98, 101]). In patients with MGD, melting point of meibomian lipids rises, which is why hot compresses, warming masks and goggles, infrared heaters, and eyelid massage led to clinical improvement with tear film stability and lipid thickness of the tear film (reduced blockage of meibomian gland excretory ducts and improvement of the meibomian secretion) [32, 54, 71, 101–103]. Tetracyclines are bacteriostatic antibiotics with anti-inflammatory effect (reduction of the synthesis and activity of matrix metalloproteinases, production of IL-1 and TNF-α, activity of collagenases and B-cell activation). A low-dose treatment for 6–12 weeks improves tear film stability, tear production, and symptoms (higher dosages are connected with higher rate of adverse events) [32, 102–105]. Macrolides (azithromycin) have both bacteriostatic and anti-inflammatory effect. They improve meibomian gland function and symptoms, reduce bacterial colonization of eyelid and normalize meibomian gland secretion [32, 106, 107].

To reduce degree of ocular surface exposure for environmental factors and for evaporation a partial closure/closure of the eyelid may be indicated: for short periods, botulinum injections have been used; in other cases, surgical procedures may be considered [28, 108].

6.10 Other therapies

6.10.1 Systemic immunomodulatory and biologic therapy

The treatment with systemic immunosuppression in patients with DED and SS requires clinical trials to assess it [2, 22, 52]. Antimalarials (hydroxychloroquine and chloroquine), in some studies, were found to have benefits for SS DED, but in others, there was no change (test Schirmer 1, FTBUT) between baseline and the end point; OSDI improved, but there was no statistical difference between treating group and placebo [2, 109–111]. Methotrexate (MTX) has well-documented efficacy in uveitis and scleritis, but there is no data that confirm it works in SS DED: one case report on improvement with MTX therapy [2, 112]. In one open-label study, improvement in symptoms but no changes in signs of DED in patients with pSS treated with mycophenolate mofetil were reported [2, 113]. Rituximab (anti-CD 20 monoclonal antibody) in some studies improved symptoms of DED, in others there was no statistical significance on the final results of ocular dryness and Schirmer 1 testing [2, 52, 114]. There was no improvement in both symptoms and signs after etanercept therapy [52, 115], abatacept (CTLA4-Ig) in some studies improved results of Schirmer 1 test, in others there were changes in FTBUT [2, 116].

6.10.2 Hormone therapy

There are some studies on the use of hormonal therapy in patients with DED. Association of low androgen levels with lacrimal gland inflammation and lacrimal insufficiency were found, consequently androgen supplementation could be a potential therapy in DED [97, 117]. Studies on systemic estrogen and estrogen-androgen therapy revealed that estrogen-only therapy may intensify ocular irritation (no benefits in symptoms and signs); however, topical estrogen therapy seems to be beneficial for DED because of the influence on ocular epithelial cells. Combined estrogen-androgen therapy improves symptoms of DED [97, 118–120]. Although dehydroepiandrosterone (DHEA) may replenish suppressed hormonal levels in pSS and improve sicca symptoms, first data on DED symptoms and signs after DHEA therapy have not revealed improvement [95, 121, 122].

6.10.3 Others

In literature, we can find some more possibilities of DED treatment in SS patients, but they are published as case reports or clinical studies. Neurostimulation of nasolacrimal pathway stimulates lacrimal gland secretion that improves scores of Schirmer I test and results of ocular staining. A new device for intranasal neurostimulation provides small electrical pulses to stimulate production of patients' tears [22, 123]. Local radiotherapy to the lacrimal gland was reported as a successful treatment in a patient with SS and lacrimal gland involvement [51, 124]. There are experimental studies on topical administration of lacritin (tear glycoprotein with prosecretory, prosurvival, and mitogenic properties) and interleukin-1 receptor antagonist—anakinra (targeting IL-1/IL-1R1 signaling pathway) in aqua-deficiency DED and both of them are promising for future [125, 126]. Therapy with oral lactoferrin (tear protein modulating oxidative stress and regulating microbes) improved corneal sensitivity compared to placebo [52, 127], as well as herbs used in traditional Chinese medicine revealed beneficial effect for symptoms and Schirmer 1 test score compared to placebo [52, 127, 128], but both methods are limited in routine clinic because of the lack of explanation of molecular mechanisms or target limits [52].

7. Conclusion

Dry eye disease is an inseparable part of the both types of Sjögren's syndrome. There is no specific test to diagnose it—for everyday practice, several tests are used to diagnose and to interpret the severity of the problem. Moreover, though it is more severe than in other diseases, there is no specific test for DED in SS.

The treatment of DED in SS is also the same as in other patients. Patients are treated with both topical and systemic therapies. There are some trials to use immunosuppressive agents for DED in SS to provide relief to eye dryness symptoms, but there are not enough verified studies on it.

Both in diagnostic and therapeutic problems of DED, there are still challenges for the future and need further multicenter, double-blind, randomized studies.

Author details

Dorota Kopacz* and Piotr Maciejewicz
Department of Ophthalmology, Medical University of Warsaw, Warsaw, Poland

*Address all correspondence to: dr.dk@wp.pl

References

[1] Utine CA, Akpek EK. What ophthalmologists should know about Sjögren's syndrome. European Ophthalmic Review. 2010;**4**:77-80

[2] Gonzales AJ, Lietman TM. Ocular involvement in Sjögren's syndrome: Advances in therapy. Current Treatment Options in Neurology. 2018;**4**:99-109

[3] Billings M, Dye BA, Iafolla T, Baer AN, Grisius M, Alevizos I. Significance and implications of patient-reported xerostomia in Sjögren's syndrome: Findings from the National Institutes of Health cohort. eBioMedicine. 2016;**12**:270-279

[4] Both T, Dalm VASH, van Hagen M, van Daele PLA. Reviewing primary Sjögren's syndrome: Beyond the dryness—From pathophysiology to diagnosis and treatment. International Journal of Medical Sciences. 2017;**14**(3):191-200

[5] Asmussen K, Andersen V, Bendixen G, Schiodt M, Oxholm P. A new model for classification of disease manifestations in primary Sjögren'ssyndrome: Evaluation in retrospective long-term study. Journal of Internal Medicine. 1996;**239**:475-482

[6] Song IS, Lee S-M. Ocular manifestation of Sjögren's syndrome. Hanyang Medical Reviews. 2016;**36**:161-167

[7] Kassan SS, Thomas TL, Moutsopoulos HM, Hoover R, et al. Increased risk of lymphoma in sicca syndrome. Annals of Internal Medicine. 1978;**89**:888-892

[8] Zufferey P, Meyer OC, Grossin M, Kahn MF. Primary Sjögren syndrome (SS) and malignant lymphoma. A retrospective cohort study of 55 patients with SS. Scandinavian Journal of Rheumatology. 1995;**24**:342-345

[9] Report of the definition and classification of the international dry eye workshop. The Ocular Surface. 2007;**5**:75-92

[10] Gupta A, Sadeghi PB, Akpek EK. Occult thyroid eye disease in patients presenting with dry eye syndrome. American Journal of Ophthalmology. 2009;**147**:919-923

[11] Ken E, Demirag MD, Beyazyildz E. Presence of Sjögren's syndrome in dry eye patients. Rheumatology (Sunnyvale). 2014;**4**(2):137

[12] Akpek EK, Klimava A, Thorne JE, Martin D, et al. Evaluation of patients with dry eye for presence of underlying Sjögren syndrome. Cornea. 2009;**28**(5):493-497

[13] Tzioufas AG, Kapsogeorgou EK, Moutsopoulos HM. Pathogenesis of Sjögren's syndrome; what we know and what we should learn. Journal of Autoimmunity. 2012;**39**:4-8

[14] Akpek EK, Gottsch JD. Immune defense at the ocular surface. Eye. 2003;**17**:949-956

[15] Barone F, Bombardieri M, Manzo A, Blades MC, et al. Association of CXCL13 and CCL21 expression with the progressive organization of lymphoid-like structures in Sjogren's syndrome. Arthritis and Rheumatism. 2005;**52**:1773-1784

[16] Darion C, Devauchelle V, Hutin P, Le Berre R, et al. Aberrant expression of BAFF by B lymphocytes infiltrating the salivary glands of patients with primary Sjögren's syndrome. Arthritis and Rheumatism. 2007;**56**:1334-1344

[17] Hansen A, Lipsky PE, Dorner T. Immunopathogenesis of primary Sjogren's syndrome: Implications for disease management and therapy.

Current Opinion in Rheumatology. 2005;**17**:558-565

[18] Pavlakis PP, Alexopoulos H, Kosmidis ML, Mamali I, et al. Peripheral neuropathies in Sjögren syndrome: A critical update on clinical features and pathogenetic mechanisms. Journal of Autoimmunity. 2012;**39**:27-33

[19] Vitali C, Bombardieri S, Moutsopoulos HM, Belestrieri G, et al. Preliminary criteria for classification of Sjögren's syndrome. Results of prospective concerted action supported by the European Community. Arthritis and Rheumatism. 1993;**36**(3):340-347

[20] Vitali C, Bombardieri S, Jonsson R, Moutsopoulos HM, et al. Classification criteria for Sjögren's syndrome: A revised version of the European criteria proposed by the American-European Consensus Group. Annals of the Rheumatic Diseases. 2002;**61**:554-558

[21] Shiboski CH, Shiboski SC, Seror R, Criswell LA, et al. 2016 American College of Rheumatology/ European League Against Rheumatism Classification Criteria for Primary Sjögren's Syndrome. A consensus and data-driven methodology involving three international patient cohorts. Arthritis & Rheumatology. 2017;**69**:35-45

[22] Kuklinski E, Asbell PA. Sjögren's syndrome from the perspective of ophthalmology. Clinical Ophthalmology. 2017;**182**:55-61

[23] Whitcher JP, Shiboski CH, Shiboski SC, Am H, et al. A simplified quantitative method for assessing keratoconjunctivitis sicca from the Sjögren's Syndrome International Registry. American Journal of Ophthalmology. 2010;**149**(3):405-415

[24] Menzies KL, Srinivasan S, Prokopich CL, Jones L. Infrared imaging of Meibomian glands and evaluation of the lipid layer in Sjögren syndrome patients and nondry eye controls. Investigative Ophthalmology & Visual Science. 2005;**56**:836-841

[25] Kassan SS, Moutsopoulos HM. Clinical manifestation and early diagnosis of Sjögren's syndrome. Archives of Internal Medicine. 2004;**164**:1275-1284

[26] Bartlett JD, Keith MS, Sudharsan L, Snedecor SJ. Association between signs and symptoms of dry eye disease: A systemic review. Clinical Ophthalmology. 2015;**9**:1719-1730

[27] Sullivan BD, Crews LA, Messmer EM, Foulks GN, et al. Correlations between commonly used objective signs and symptoms for the diagnosis of dry eye disease: Clinical implications. Acta Ophthalmologica. 2014;**92**:161-166

[28] Foulks GN, Forstot SL, Donshik PC, Forstot JZ, et al. Clinical guidelines for management of dry eye associated with Sjögren disease. The Ocular Surface. 2015;**13**:118-132

[29] Schaumberg DA, Sullivan DA, Buring JE, Dana MR. Prevalence of dry eye syndrome among US women. American Journal of Ophthalmology. 2003;**136**:318-326

[30] Schaumberg DA, Dana MR, Buring JE, Sullivan DA. Prevalence of dry eye disease among US men: Estimates from the Physicians' Health Studies. Archives of Ophthalmology. 2009;**127**:763-768

[31] Oden NL, Lilienfeld DE, Lemp MA, Nelson JD, et al. Sensitivity and specificity of a screening questionnaire for dry eye. Advances in Experimental Medicine and Biology. 1998;**438**:807-820

[32] Messmer EM. The pathophysiology, diagnosis and treatment of dry eye disease. Deutsches Ärzteblatt International. 2015;**112**:71-82

[33] Goto T, Zheng Z, Okamoto S, Ohashi Y. Tear film stability analysis system: Introducing a new application for videokeratography. Cornea. 2004;**23**(8supp):S56-S70

[34] Gumus K, Crockett CH, Rao K, Yeu E, et al. Noninvasive assessment of tear stability with the tear stability analysis system in tear dysfunction patients. Investigative Ophthalmology & Visual Science. 2011;**52**(1):456-461

[35] Kim M, Kim HS, Na K-S. Correlation between tear osmolarity and other ocular surface parameters in primary Sjögren syndrome. Korean Journal of Ophthalmology. 2017;**31**(1):25-31

[36] Ng ALK, Choy BNK, Chan TCY, Wong IYH, et al. Comparison of tear osmolarity in rheumatoid arthritis patients with and without secondary Sjögren syndrome. Cornea. 2017;**36**(7):805-809

[37] Utine CA, Bicakcigil M, Yavuz S, Ciftci F. Tera osmolarity measurements in dry eye related to primary Sjögren's syndrome. Current Eye Research. 2011;**36**:683-690

[38] Bunya VY, Langelier N, Chen S, Pistilli M, et al. Tear osmolarity in patients with Sjogren syndrome. Cornea. 2013;**32**:922-927

[39] Dastjerdi MH, Dana R. Corneal nerve alterations in dry eye-associated ocular surface disease. International Ophthalmology Clinics. 2009;**49**:11-20

[40] Zhao H, Li Q, Ye M, Yu J. Tera Luminex anlysisi in dry eye patients. Medical Science Monitor. 2018;**24**:7595-7602

[41] Tong L, Wong TY, Cheng Y. Level of tear cytokines in population-level participants and correlation with clinical features. Cytokine. 2018;**110**:452-458

[42] Nelson JD, Shimazaki JM, Benitez-del-Castillo, Craig JP, et al. The international workshop on Meibomian gland dysfunction: Report of the definition and classification subcommittee. Investigative Ophthalmology & Visual Science. 2011;**52**:933-939

[43] Goto E, Matsumoto Y, Kamoi M, Endo K, et al. Tear evaporation rates in Sjogren syndrome and non-Sjogren dry eye patients. American Journal of Ophthalmology. 2007;**144**:81-85

[44] Bron AJ, Tiffany JM, Gouveia SM, Yokoi N, et al. Functional aspects of the tear film lipid layer. Experimental Eye Research. 2004;**78**:374-360

[45] Finis D, Pischel N, Schrader S, Geerling G. Evaluation of lipid layer thickness measurements of the tear film as diagnostic tool for Meibomian gland disfunction. Cornea. 2003;**32**:1549-1553

[46] Jung JW, Park SY, Kim JS, Kim EK, et al. Analysis of factors associated with the tear film lipid layer thickness in normal eyes and patients with dry eye syndrome. Investigative Ophthalmology & Visual Science. 2016;**57**:4076-4083

[47] Ji YW, Lee J, Lee H, Seo KY, et al. Automated measurements of tear film dynamics and lipid layer thickness for assessment of non-Sjogren dry eye syndrome with Meibomian gland dysfunction. Cornea. 2017;**36**:176-182

[48] Best N, Drury L, Wolffsohn JS. Clinical evaluation of the oculus keratograph. Contact Lens & Anterior Eye. 2012;**35**:171-174

[49] The Oculus Keratograph ® 5M Software. Arlington, WA: Oculus Inc. Available at: https://www.oculus.de/us/products/topography/keratography-5m/software/tf-scan/#producte-navi

[50] Rodriges JD, Johnson PR, Ousler GW 3rd, Smith LM, et al. Automated

grading system for evaluation of ocular redness associated with dry eye. Clinical Ophthalmology. 2013;**7**:1197-1204

[51] Herzlich A, Aquavella JV. Ophthalmologic manifestations of Sjogren syndrome. Available from: https://emedicine.medscape.com/article/1192919

[52] Villani E, Galimberti D, Viola F, Mapelli C, et al. The cornea in Sjogren's syndrome: An in vivo confocal study. Investigative Ophthalmology & Visual Science. 2007;**48**(5):2017-2022

[53] Shih KC, Lun CN, Jhanji V, Thong BY-H, et al. Systemic review of randomized controlled trials in the treatment of dry eye disease in Sjogren syndrome. Journal of Inflammation. 2017;**14**:26. DOI: 10.1186/s12950-017-0174-3

[54] Management and therapy for dry eye disease: Report of the Management and Therapy Subcommittee of the International Dry Eye Workshop. The Ocular Surface. 2007;**5**:163-178

[55] Galperi G, Berra M, Marquez MI, Mandaradoni M, et al. Impact of environmental pollution on the ocular surface of Sjögren's syndrome patients. Arquivos Brasileiros de Oftalmologia. 2018;**81**(6):481-489

[56] Luo L, Li DQ, Corrales RM, Pflugfelder SC. Hyperosmolar saline is a proinflammatory stress on the mouse ocular surface. Eye & Contact Lens. 2005;**31**:186-193

[57] Lee SY, Tong L. Lipid-containing lubricants for dry eye: A systemic review. Optometry and Vision Science. 2012;**89**:1654-1661

[58] Messmer EM. Preservatives in ophthalmology. Der Ophthalmologe. 2012;**109**:1064-1070

[59] Wander AH, Koffler BH. Extending the duration of tear film protection in dry eye syndrome: Review and retrospective case series study of the hydroxypropyl cellulose ophthalmic insert. The Ocular Surface. 2009;**7**:154-162

[60] Hong S, Kim T, Chung SH, Kim EK, et al. Recurrence after topical nonpreserved methylprednisolone therapy for keratoconjunctivitis sicca in Sjögren's syndrome. Journal of Ocular Pharmacology and Therapeutics. 2007;**23**:78-82

[61] Lin T, Gong L. Topical fluorometholone treatment for ocular dryness in patients with Sjogren syndrome. A randomized clinical trial in China. Medicine (Baltimore). 2015;**94**(7):e551. DOI: 10.1097/MD.0000000000000551

[62] Aragona P, Spinalla R, Rania L, Postorino E, et al. Safety and efficacy of 0.1% clobetasone butyrate eyedrops in the treatment of dry eye in Sjögren syndrome. European Journal of Ophthalmology. 2013;**23**(3):368-376

[63] Lee HK, Fyu IH, Seo KY, Hong S, et al. Topical 0.1% prednisolone lowers nerve growth factor expression in keratoconjunctivitis sicca patients. Ophthalmology. 2006;**113**:198-205

[64] Marsh P, Pflugfeld SC. Topical nonpreserved methylprednisolone therapy for keratoconjunctivitis sicca in Sjogren syndrome. Ophthalmology. 1999;**106**:811-816

[65] Waldmeier Zimmermann K, Qian T, Tintelnot-Blomey M, et al. Cyclophilin D as a drug target. Current Medicinal Chemistry. 2003;**10**(16):1485-1506

[66] Othman TM, Mousa A, Gikandi PW, AbdelMabod M, et al. Efficacy and safety of using topical cyclosporine A for treatment of moderate to severe dry eye disease. Saudi J Ophthalmol. 2018;**32**:217-221

[67] Sall K, Stevenson OD, Mundorf TK, Reis BL. Two multicenter, randomized studies of the efficacy of cyclosporine ophthalmic emultion in moderate to severe dry eye disease. CsA Phase 3 Study Group. Ophthalmology. 2000;**107**(4):631-639

[68] Kunert KS, Tisdale AS, Stern ME, Smith JA, et al. Analysis of topical cyclosporine treatment of patients with dry eye syndrome: Effect on conjunctival lymphocytes. Archives of Ophthalmology. 2000;**118**(11):1489-1496

[69] Yoshida A, Fujihara T, Nakata K. Cyclosporin A increases tear fluid secretion via release of sensory neurotransmitters and muscarinic pathway in mice

[70] Perry HD, Donnenfeld ED. Topical 0.05% cyclosporin in the treatment of dry eye. Expert Opinion on Pharmacotherapy. 2004;**5**:2099-2107

[71] Geerling G, Tauber J, Bauduin C, Goto E, et al. The international workshopmeibomian gland dysfunction: Report of the subcommittee on management and treatment of meibomian gland dysfunction. Investigative Ophthalmology & Visual Science. 2011;**52**(4):2050-2064

[72] Perry HD, Doshi-Carnevale S, Donnenfeld ED, Solomon R, et al. Efficacy of commercially available topical cyclosporine A 0.05% in the treatment of meibomian gland dysfunction. Cornea. 2006;**25**(2):171-175

[73] Rubin M, Rao SN. Efficacy of topical cyclosporine A 0.05%in the treatment of posterior blepharitis. Journal of Ocular Pharmacology and Therapeutics. 2006;**22**(10):47-53

[74] Barber LD, Pflugfelder SC, Tauber J, Foulks GN. Phase 3 safety evaluation of cyclosporine 0.1% ophthalmic emultion administrated twice daily to dry eye disease patients for up to 3 years. Ophthalmology. 2005;**112**:1790-1794

[75] Abidi A, Shukla P, Ahmad A. Liftegrast: A novel drug for treatment of dry eye disease. Journal of Pharmacology and Pharmacotherapeutics. 2016;**7**(4):194-198

[76] Tauber J, Karpecki PM, Latkany R, Luchs J, et al. Lifitegrast ophthalmic solution 5.0% versus placebo for treatment of dry eye disease: Results of the randomized phase III OPUS-2 study. Ophthalmology. 2015;**122**(12):2423-2431

[77] Nichols KK, Holland E, Toyos MM, Peace JH, et al. Ocular comfort assessment of lifitegrast ophthalmic solution 5.0% in OPUs-3, a phase III randomized controlled trial. Clinical Ophthalmology. 2018;**12**:263-270

[78] Holland E, Luchs J, Karpecki PM, Nichols KK, et al. Lifitegrast for the treatment of dry eye disease: Results of a Phase III, randomized, double-masked, placebo-controlled trial (OPUS-3). Ophthalmology. 2017;**124**(1):53-60

[79] Lollett IV, Galor A. Dry eye syndrome: Developments and lifitegrast in perspective. Clinical Ophthalmology. 2018;**12**:125-139

[80] Semeraro F, Forbice E, Nascimbeni G, Taglietti M, et al. Effect of autologous serum eye drops in patients with Sjogren syndrome-related dry eye: Clinical and in vivo confocal microscopy evaluation of the ocular surface. In Vivo. 2016;**30**:931-938

[81] Tananuvat N, Daniell M, Sullivan LJ, Yi Q, et al. Controlled study of the use of autologous serum in dry eye patients. Cornea. 2001;**20**:802-806

[82] Kojima T, Ishida R, Dogru M, Gotu E, et al. The effect of autologous serum

eyedrops in the treatment of severe dry eye disease: A prospective randomized case-control study. American Journal of Ophthalmology. 2005;**139**:242-246

[83] Urzua CA, Vasquez DH, Huidobro A, Hernandez H, et al. Randomized double-blind clinical trial of autologous serum versus artificial tears in dry eye syndrome. Current Eye Research. 2012;**37**(8):684-688

[84] Lopez-Plandolit S, Morales MC, Freire V, Grau AE, et al. Efficacy of plasma rich in growth factors for the treatment of dry eye. Cornea. 2011;**30**(12):1312-1317

[85] Alio JL, Colecha JR, Pastor S, Rodrigez Z, et al. Treatment of dry eye disease with autologous platelet-rich plasma: A prospective, interventional, non-randomized study. Ophthalmology and therapy. 2017;**6**:285-293

[86] Lopez-Plandolit S, Morales MC, Freire V, Etxebarria J, et al. Plasma rich in growth factors as a therapeutic agent for persistent corneal epithelial defects. Cornea. 2010;**29**(8):843-848

[87] Tandon A, Tovey JC, Sharma A, Gupta R, et al. Role of transforming growth factor beta in corneal function, biology and pathology. Current Molecular Medicine. 2010;**10**(6):565-578

[88] Tsifetaki N, Kitsos G, Pashides C, et al. Oral pilocarpine for the treatment of ocular symptoms in patients with Sjogren syndrome: A randomized 12 week controlled study. Annals of the Rheumatic Diseases. 2003;**62**:1204-1207

[89] Aragona P, Di Pietro R, Spinella R, Mobrici M. Conjunctival epithelium improvement after systemic pilocarpine in patients with Sjogren syndrome. The British Journal of Ophthalmology. 2006;**90**:166-170

[90] Ono M, Takamura E, Schinozkai K, et al. Therapeutic effect of cevimeline on dry eye in patients with Sjogren syndrome: A randomized, double-blind study. American Journal of Ophthalmology. 2004;**138**:6-17

[91] Fezza JP. Cross-linked hyaluronic acid gel occlusive device for the treatment of dry eye syndrome. Clinical Ophthalmology. 2018;**12**:2277-2283

[92] Foulds WS. Intracanalicular gelatin implants in the treatment of keratoconjunctivitis sicca. The British Journal of Ophthalmology. 1961;**45**:625-627

[93] Freeman JM. The punctum plug: Evaluation of a new treatment for the dry eye. Transactions – American Academy of Ophthalmology and Otolaryngology. 1975;**79**:OP874-OP879

[94] Qui W, Liu Z, Ao M, et al. Punctal plugs versus artificial tears for treating primary Sjogren syndrome with keratoconjunctivitis sicca: A comparative observation of their effects on visual function. Rheumatology International. 2013;**33**:2543-2548

[95] Russo PA, Bouchaard CS, Galasso JM. Extended-wear silicone hydrogel soft contact lenses in the management of moderate to severe dry eye signs and symptoms secondary to graft-versus-host disease. Eye & Contact Lens. 2007;**33**:144-147

[96] Pallum K, Buckley R. Therapeutic and ocular surface indication for scleral contact lenses. The Ocular Surface. 2007;**5**:40-48

[97] Foulks GN. Treatment of dry eye disease by the non-ophthalmologist. Rheumatic Diseases Clinics of North America. 2008;**34**:987-1000

[98] Rashid S, Jin Y, Ecoiffier T, Barabino S, et al. Topical omega-3 and omega-6 acids for treatment of dry eye. Archives of Ophthalmology. 2008;**126**(2):219-225

[99] Calder PC, Zurier RB. Polyunstructurated fatty acids and rheumatoid arthritis. Current Opinion in Clinical Nutrition and Metabolic Care. 2001;**4**(2):115-121

[100] Aragona P, Bucolo C, Spinella R, Giuffrida S, et al. Systemic omega-6 essential fatty acid treatment and pge-1 tear content in Sjögren's syndrome patients. Investigative Ophthalmology & Visual Science. 2005;**46**(12):4474-4479

[101] Kim MJ, Stinnet SS, Gupta PK. Effect of thermal pulsation treatment on tear film parameters in dry eye disease patients. Clinical Ophthalmology. 2017;**11**:883-886

[102] Guillon M, Maissa C, Wong S. Eyelid margin modification associated with eyelid hygiene in anterior blepharitis and Meibomian gland dysfunction. Eye & Contact Lens. 2012;**38**:319-325

[103] Urslow C. Evaluation of the ocular tolerance of novel eyelid-warming device used for Meibomian gland dysfunction. Contact Lens & Anterior Eye. 2013;**36**:226-231

[104] Solomon A, Rosenblatt M, Li DQ, Liu Z, et al. Doxycycline inhibition of interleukin-1 in the corneal epithelium. Investigative Ophthalmology & Visual Science. 2000;**41**:2544-2557

[105] Smith VA, Cook SD. Doxycycline—A role in ocular surface repair. The British Journal of Ophthalmology. 2004;**88**:619-625

[106] Sadrai Z, Hajrasouliha AR, Chauhan S, Saban DR, et al. Effect of topical azithromycin on corneal innate immune response. Investigative Ophthalmology & Visual Science. 2011;**52**:2525-2531

[107] Haque RM, Torkildsen GL, Brubaker K, Zink RC, et al. Multicenter open-label study evaluating the efficacy of azithromycin ophthalmic solution 1% on the signs and symptoms of subjects with blepharitis. Cornea. 2010;**29**:871-877

[108] Benvenuti D. Botox use in prevention of dry eyes. Plastic and Reconstructive Surgery. 1998;**102**(3):918

[109] Both T, Dalm VA, van Hagen PM, Van Daele PL. Reviewing primary Sjogren's syndrome: Beyond the dryness—From the pathophysiology to diagnosis and treatment. International Journal of Medical Sciences. 2017;**14**:191-200

[110] Yavuz S, Asfuroglu E, Bicakcigil M, Toker E. Hydroxychloroquine improve dry eye syndrome of patients with primary Sjogren's syndrome. Rheumatology International. 2011;**31**:1045-1049

[111] Fox RI, Dixon R, Guarrasi V, Krubel S. Treatment of primary Sjogren's syndrome with hydroxychloroquine: A retrospective open-label study. Lupus. 1996;**5**(suppl. 1):S31-S36

[112] Cordero-Coma M, Anzaar F, Sorbin L, Foster CS. Systemic immunomodulatory therapy in severe dry eye secondary to inflammation. Ocular Immunology and Inflammation. 2007;**15**:99-104

[113] Willeke P, Schlüter B, Becker H, Schotte H, et al. Mycophenolate sodium treatment in patients with primary Sjogren syndrome: A pilot trial. Arthritis Research & Therapy. 2007;**9**(6):R115

[114] Devauchelle-Pensec V, Mariette X, Jousse-Joulin S, Berthelot JM, et al. Treatment of primary Sjogren syndrome with rituximab: A randomized trial. Annals of Internal Medicine. 2014;**160**:233-242

[115] Sankar V, Brennan MT, Kok MR, Leakan RA, et al. Etanercept in Sjogren's

syndrome: A twelve-week randomized, double-blind, placebo-controlled pilot clinical trial. Arthritis and Rheumatism. 2004;**50**(7):2240-2245

[116] Meiner PM, Vissink A, Kroese FGM, Spijkervet FKL, et al. Abatacept treatment reduces disease activity in early primary Sjogren's syndrome (open-label proof of concept ASAP study). Annals of the Rheumatic Diseases. 2014;**73**:1393-1396

[117] Sullivan DA. Sex hormones and Sjogren 's syndrome. The Journal of Rheumatology. 1997;**24**:17-32

[118] Schaumbegr DA, Buring JE, Sullivan DA, et al. Hormone replacement therapy and dry eye syndrome. JAMA. 2001;**286**(17):2114-2119

[119] Nascent Pharmaceuticals. iDestrin estradiol. www.nascentpharma.com

[120] Scott G, Yiu SC, Wasilewski D, Song J, et al. Combined esterified estrogen and methyltestosterone treatment for dry eye syndrome in postmenopausal woman. American Journal of Ophthalmology. 2005;**139**:1109-1110

[121] Forsblad-d'Elia H, Carlsten H, Labrie F, Konttinen YT, et al. Low serum levels of sex steroids are associated with disease characteristics in primary Sjogren's syndrome; supplementation with dehydrospiandrosterone restores the concentrations. Journal of Clinical Endocrinology & Metabolism. 2009;**94**(6):2044-2051

[122] Pillemer SR, Brennan MT, Sankar V, Leaken RA, et al. Pilot clinical trial of dehydrospiandrosterone (DHEA) versus placebo for Sjogren's syndrome. Arthritis and Rheumatism. 2004;**51**(4):601-614

[123] Hillman L. Neurostimulation offers a new frontier in dry eye treatment. Source. https://www.eyeworld.org/

[124] Patera J, Sirak I, Langrova H, Maisnar V et al. Successful radiotherapy treatment of lacrimal gland infiltration inpatients with and without Sjogren's syndrome. Bratislavské Lekárske Listy. 2012;**11394**:249-250

[125] Vijmasi T, Chen FYT, Balasubbu S, Gallup M, et al. Topical administration of lacritin is a novel therapy for aqueous-deficient dry eye disease. Investigative Ophthalmology & Visual Science. 2014;**55**:5401-5409

[126] Vijmasi T, Chen FYT, Chen YT, Gallup M, et al. Topical administration of interleukin-1 receptor antagonist as a therapy for aqueous-deficient dry eye in autoimmune disease. Molecular Vision. 2013;**19**:1957-1965

[127] Dogru M, Massumoto Y, Yamamoto Y, Goto E, et al. Lactoferrin in Sjogren's syndrome. Ophthalmology. 2007;**114**(12):2366-2367

[128] Hu W, Quian X, Guo F, Zhang M, et al. Traditional Chinese medicine compound Sheng Jin Run Zao Yang Xue granules for treatment of primary Sjogren's syndrome; a randomized, double-blind, placebo controlled trial. Chinese Medical Journal. 2014;**127**(15):2721-2726

Chapter 4

Laryngological and Dental Manifestations of Sjögren's Syndrome

Bartłomiej Kamiński and Katarzyna Błochowiak

Abstract

Sjögren's syndrome (SS) affects numerous different areas, and many specialists may be involved in the diagnosis and treatment of SS. Otolaryngological and dental manifestations, neurological impairment, and hearing loss may be the initial symptoms of SS. This chapter describes the most common otolaryngological and oral manifestations of SS, its pathomechanism and possible etiology. Dryness accompanying SS is associated with many clinical implications. The rate of dry mouth in SS ranged from 41% at initial diagnosis to 84% 10 years after diagnosis. An unstimulated salivary flow rate of 0.1 ml/min in sialometry gives a score of 1 to the weighted sum of 5 items according to the current EULAR/ACR criteria. The presence of mononuclear cell aggregates around the ducts and acini of salivary glands results in functional and structural alterations at the level of these glands and impairs their secretory function. The most common oral signs and symptoms are dental caries, tooth decay, fungal infections, traumatic oral lesions, dysphagia, dysgeusia, and inflammation of the salivary glands. Saliva in SS is characterized by the increased concentration of lactoferrin, potassium and cystatin C and the decreased concentration of amylase, carbonic anhydrase, mucins, histatines, IgA, statherins, proline-rich proteins, and the loss of salivary buffer properties. The lack of these physiological defense mechanisms increases the risk of opportunistic infections, mainly fungal infections by *Candida albicans*. Candidiasis accompanies angular cheilitis, simple cheilitis, and exfoliative cheilitis. The salivary glands of SS patients are characterized by chronic inflammation with the presence of lymphocytic infiltrates located around the striated ducts. These periductal foci may lead to the development of organized ectopic lymphoid structures resembling secondary lymphoid organs with segregated T- and B-cell areas, and high endothelial venules. These structures become an active center of immune response. The presence of foci in labial salivary glands is a hallmark of SS, and their histopathologic analysis is an important item in the diagnosis and classification. A biopsy can be taken from either the labial or the parotid salivary gland, but currently according to the diagnostic criteria, only labial salivary gland biopsy (LSGB) is recommended to confirm the diagnosis of SS. The authors present their own experience and recommendations in taking labial salivary gland biopsy, the main surgical approaches, and the main limitations for this diagnostic method and describe the possibilities and principles of histopathological examination in SS. The authors present the main ultrasonic signs of SS major salivary glands and perspectives of the usage of salivary gland ultrasonic examination in the diagnosis and monitoring of SS. The presented chapter also includes the most common laryngological manifestations associated with SS: nose dryness, crusting, or atrophy of the nasal mucosa, dryness of the throat, dysphagia, hoarseness, otalgia and tinnitus, gastro-esophageal reflux, and chronic cough. Patients with SS tend to have a higher prevalence of sensorineural hearing impairment compared with the general population. Idiopathic hearing loss may represent the initial manifestation of SS. Furthermore, authors present and discuss the main neurological symptoms of SS. Neurological manifestations are reported in about 20% of patients with SS. In patients with SS, neurological manifestations may occur, such as peripheral neuropathy and other forms of neuropathies, including sensory ataxia, painful sensory neuropathy without sensory ataxia, multiple mononeuropathy, multiple cranial neuropathy, autonomic neuropathy, radiculoneuropathy and intra- and extraoral paresthesias, facial hypaesthesia, and trigeminal nerve neuropathy.

Keywords: Sjögren's syndrome, hearing loss, cranial nerve neuropathy, xerostomia

1. Introduction

Microscopic findings involving lymphocytic infiltration surrounding the excretory ducts in combination with the destruction of acinar tissue are representative for both minor and major salivary glands and are pathognomonic changes for SS. Parotid, lip, or sublingual salivary gland biopsy is performed in the diagnosis and monitoring of SS, but currently only labial salivary gland biopsy (LSGB) is included into classification criteria of SS. LSGB is used for the diagnosis of Sjögren's syndrome (SS). The current classification criteria of SS, approved by the American College of Rheumatology (ACR) and the European League against Rheumatism (EULAR) in 2016, include LSGB as a part of weighted sum of five items [1]. The presence of focal lymphocytic sialadenitis (FLS) with a focus score of 1 foci/4 mm^2 glandular tissue is a positive score of LSGB. Lip salivary glands are widely distributed in the labial mucosa of the oral cavity. They are largely used for assisting the diagnosis of SS, because they are easily accessible and lie above the muscle layer. They are separated from the oral mucous membrane by a thin layer of fibrous connective tissue. Orientation and identification of glandular tissue is the easiest. The risk of excessive postoperative bleeding is decreased because the arterial supply to the lip lies deep. These anatomical implications and pathognomic changes predispose of labial salivary glands to the biopsy [1–7].

2. Surgical technique and possible complications of LSGB

Labial salivary gland biopsy is considered a minor surgical procedure and can be performed on the ambulatory basis. There is no standardized technique that yields adequate tissue for analysis and minimizes adverse effects. The lack of uniformity in methodology and potential adverse effects of LSGB hinders its application. LSGB is treated as a safe and simple surgical procedure without severe postoperative complications. One of the most severe complications of LSGB is sensitive nerve injury. This localized sensory alternation can be described as an anesthesia, a reduced or partial loss of sensation, a transitory numbness, or a hypoesthesia. These sensations can last for a few months or can be permanent. Persistent lip numbness occurs in up to 6% of biopsies performed in the lower lip [8]. The branches of the mental nerve in the lower lip are closely associated with the salivary glands, and this anatomical relationship increases the risk of postoperative sensory sensations. Additionally, the branch of the mental nerve usually divides into two sub-branches: a horizontal and a vertical, which have an ascending course toward the vermillion border and are in close relation to the labial salivary glands. Incisional biopsies shorter than 2 cm performed with a scalpel have reported complications ranging from 0 to 9.3%, whereas those using larger incisions (2–3 cm) have described complications in the range of 3.7–31%. Transient disorders of lip sensitivity are found to occur in up to 11.7% of procedures. Persistent lower lip hypoesthesia is reported in about 3.4–4% of cases. Larger incisional biopsies and punch biopsies are associated with a higher risk of both transient and persistent lower lip numbness. Other possible complications of LSGB are less severe, usually transient or temporary, and are associated with localized postoperative inflammation or improper healing. The symptoms of postoperative inflammations are local pain and swelling. Blood vessel injuries result in hematoma. The possible delayed complications are the formation of granulomas, internal scarring, and cheloid formation. Labial salivary gland injuries can result in mucous extravasation cysts. Some patients can report burning or tingling sensations, and functional deficits during the immediate postbiopsy period such as eating, sleeping, or speech difficulties [9–12].

Labial glands biopsy may be an excisional or incisional technique. The most recommended site is normal-appearing mucosa of the lower lip. Usually, it is a scalpel biopsy. A wide range of surgical approaches have been described for harvesting a few accessory glands from the lower lip using different instruments such as a scalpel, a punch, or cup forceps. The use of a forceps with a fenestrated active end to stabilize the lip has also been suggested. The excisional biopsy is carried out by excising an ellipse of oral mucous membrane down to the muscle layer. Ideally, 6–8 minor glands must be harvested and sent for histopathologic examination. The wound should be closed with 4-0 silk sutures, which are removed after 4–5 days. The modification of this method is the technique with a mucosal excision of 3.0 × 0.75 cm. Another recommended technique is a 1.0–1.5-cm-wedge-shaped excision of the mucosa between the midline and commissure. The incisional biopsy is described as a 1.5–2.0-cm linear incision of mucosa, parallel to the vermillion border and lateral to the midline. Gorson and Ropper reported a 1-cm vertical incision just behind the wet line through the mucosa and submucosa [31]. It is usually that case that the lateral lip compartments are advocated for biopsy, because of the glandular-free zone in the center of the lower lip. Berquin et al. described an oblique incision, starting 1.5 cm from the midline and proceeding latero-inferiorly to avoid the central glandular-free zone. The vertical incision technique is associated with less pain, less swelling, less scar formation, and less difficulty in eating when compared with the horizontal incision technique. There is insufficient evidence to support the superiority of one technique over the others, and the shape and the size of the incision can be considered a matter of preference. The incision shape includes elliptical, circular, linear, horizontal, vertical, and wedge shapes, and the incision length varies from a few millimeters to 2 cm.

Another recommended modification is using loupe operation glasses to precisely excise the salivary glands without disturbing the direct underlying sensible nerves. The alternative technique to scalpel biopsy is the minor salivary gland punch biopsy. This biopsy can be performed by a single operator, and it is less expensive than classical scalpel biopsy. This technique consists of obtaining the biopsy from the buccal side of the lower lip, which is stabilized by the patient him/herself using a 4–5 mm punch, which permits the retrieval of a cylinder of tissue up to 8 mm in length. The punch biopsy is suggested because of the absence of risk to the patient and because of its simplicity. However, the punch biopsies do not provide enough material for the diagnosis of Sjögren's syndrome. Moreover, the findings of this study strongly discouraged the punch technique for minor salivary gland lip biopsy and provided information on the superiority of the linear incisional biopsy in terms of neural damage [12–16].

Based on our own clinical experience, a 1.0–1.5-cm linear, horizontal incision of mucosa parallel to the vermillion border and lateral to the midline with the tip of a 15 scalpel is worth to recommend. The lower lip should be retracted and everted under tension to expose the inner surface and allow visualization of the minor salivary glands just to the depth of the mucosa. Local anesthesia injected submucosally with 0.5–1.0 ml of 1% lidocaine with 1:200,000 epinephrine is sufficient. The anesthesia hydrodissects and lifts the mucosa away from the salivary glands, provides delivery of local anesthetic directly to sensory nerve fibers, and temporarily displaces small vessels deep in the glands to promote hemostasis and visualization during the dissection. In this technique, both margins of incision should be gently crafted to access the submucosal layer. This stage of procedure can be performed using blunt-tipped iris scissors or a scalpel by spreading in a plane perpendicular to the mucosal incision and parallel to the direction of the sensory nerve fibers. This technique is fast, simple, and leaves a small scar. The linear incision secures a good adherence of wound margins and proper and fast healing. Unfortunately, this method is not effective in small amounts of salivary glands. Sometimes, it is difficult to find the sufficient amount of labial glands. Moreover, it may be difficult to harvest a sufficient number of labial salivary glands in atrophic mucosa of patients with long-standing SS. In these cases, the recommended method is a 1-cm lenticular incision of mucosa, lateral to the midline, and removal of the mucosa to uncover the submucosal layer and obtain a few adjacent salivary glands. This technique ensures good visibility into the operating field to avoid blood vessels and nerve injures. This incision provides adequate glandular tissue for diagnosis. The wound should be closed by a few nonresorbable, single, interrupted stitches. One very important issue is to harvest only labial salivary glands without muscular or other tissues. It is the most valuable specimen for histopathological examination, because it only includes glandular tissue. Additionally, this technique decreases the risk of nerve damage and postoperative pain and assures successful healing. Sensory nerve fibers are almost always visible just below the plane of dissection, and care should be taken to identify and preserve them. The next very important issue is not to puncture the labial glands to reduce the risk of mucous extravasation cyst formation. It is even better to remove all visible labial salivary glands from the operating field before suturing in order not to damage the glands or their ducts. Patients should also avoid taking steroids before the biopsy. The factors potentially contributing to a false-negative rate include the use of oral steroids that may result in immunosuppression and confound histopathologic results. The tissue specimens should be immediately placed in a wide-mouthed container, coded, and fixed in a generous amount of 10% formalin buffered saline for 24 h (**Figures 1** and **2**).

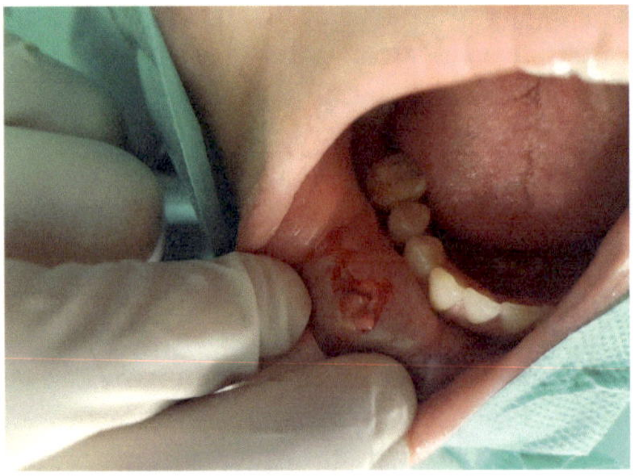

Figure 1.
Linear incision and scalpel biopsy of labial salivary gland biopsy. A few labial salivary glands exposed and visible in the operating field.

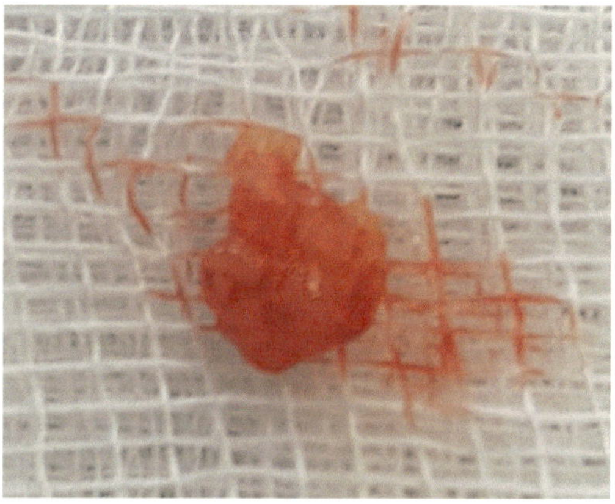

Figure 2.
Labial salivary gland specimen.

3. Histologic criteria for diagnosis of SS on labial salivary gland biopsies

Labial salivary gland biopsy is an objective test of SS and plays a significant role in the diagnostic process. In fact, the presence of either anti-SSA/SSB seropositivity or a positive lip biopsy is a requirement for an individual to be classified as having SS. The microscopic confirmation of SS is based on the presence of focal lymphocytic sialadenitis (FLS) with a focus score ≥ 1 per 4 mm^2 of glandular tissue. According to the revised American-European Consensus Group's (AECG) classification criteria and the ACR classification criteria for SS, an LSGB is considered positive if minor salivary glands demonstrate FLS, with a focus score of 1 or more, as evaluated by an expert histopathologist. A lymphocytic focus is defined as a dense aggregate of 50 or more lymphocytes adjacent to normal-appearing mucous acini in salivary gland lobules that lacked ductal dilatation. Focal lymphocytic sialadenitis is applied to specimens that show the presence of 1 or more foci of lymphocytes located in periductal and perivascular locations. The foci can contain plasma cells, but these must be a minority constituent of the inflammatory infiltrate. The focus score can be calculated for those specimens showing the histopathologic appearance of FLS. The number of lymphocytic foci is then determined for all the gland lobules in a single tissue section. The focus score is then calculated as the number of foci per square millimeter of glandular tissue multiplied by four, which then yields foci/4mm^2. A focus score of 1 equates to 1 focus/4 mm^2. To determine the focus, a calibrated eyepiece grid or image analysis software with a closed polygon tool is used. FLS has to be distinguished from nonspecific chronic sialadenitis. The symptoms of nonspecific sialadenitis are mild to moderate acinar atrophy, interstitial fibrosis, and ductal dilatation, with lymphocytes and macrophages often scattered in the parenchyma, but not forming dense aggregates of 50 or more lymphocytes immediately adjacent to normal-appearing acini. In addition to the focus score (FS), two scoring systems for salivary glands are in use for the diagnosis and classification of SS. These systems are based on the presence of foci [7]. Grading according to Tarpley's system involves destruction of acinar tissue and fibrosis (**Table 1**). Grading according to the Chisholm and Mason system is based on the presence of infiltrates from slight to one or more foci (**Table 2**) [16, 17].

Focus: a cluster of 50 or more lymphocytes and histiocytes.

Aggregate: approximately 50 cells (lymphocytes, plasma cells, or histiocytes).

Grade	Description
0	Normal
1	1 or 2 Aggregates
2	>3 Aggregates
3	Diffuse infiltrate with partial destruction of acinar tissue with or without fibrosis
4	Diffuse infiltrate with or without fibrosis destroying the lobular architecture completely

Table 1.
Grading systems for salivary gland biopsies of Tarpley.

Grade	Description
0	Absent
1	Slight infiltrate
2	Moderate infiltrate or less than one focus
3	One focus
4	More than one focus

Table 2.
Grading systems for salivary gland biopsies of Chisholm and Mason.

4. Differentiation of focus lymphocytic sialadenitis

Focus lymphocytic sialadenitis should be differentiated with other microscopic findings:

- Nonspecific chronic sialadenitis NSCS
- Sclerosing chronic sialadenitis SCS
- Granulomatous inflammation
- Infiltrates within normal limits
- Marginal zone (MALT) lymphoma
- Germinal center

Nonspecific chronic sialadenitis (NSCN) is characterized by scattered or focal infiltrates of lymphocytes, macrophages, and plasma cells that are not adjacent to normal-appearing acini and located in gland lobules that exhibit some combination of acinar atrophy, interstitial fibrosis, duct dilation, and luminal inspissated mucus.

Sclerosing chronic sialadenitis (SCS) is an advanced stage of NSCS in which interstitial fibrosis, various patterns of chronic inflammation, and acinar atrophy predominate.

Granulomatous inflammation is present when there are clusters of CD68 positive macrophages, with or without occasional multinucleated giant cells and absent necrosis.

Infiltrates within normal limits can be diagnosed in minor salivary glands with normal appearing architecture and scattered plasma cells, but without acinar atrophy and few if any lymphocytes.

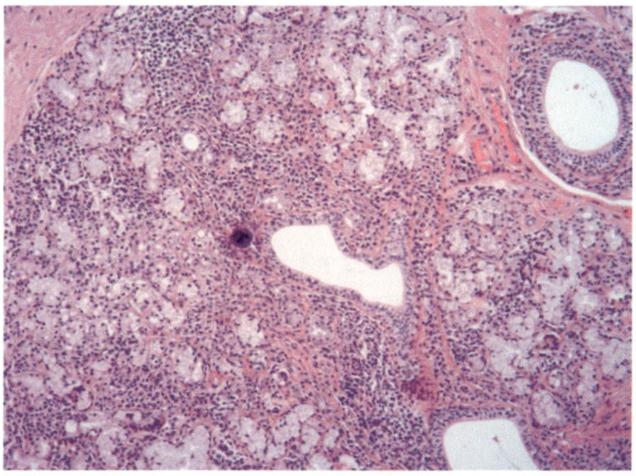

Figure 3.
Confirmation of SS in LSGB. Focus score 4 (staining H&E, magnitude 10×).

Marginal zone (MALT) lymphoma is diagnosed in minor salivary glands exhibiting diffuse lymphocytic infiltration with loss of glandular architecture and composed of sheets of CD20 positive cells without follicular distribution, few scattered CD3 positive cells, and few if any follicular dendritic (CD21 or CD23 positive) cells.

Germinal center presence is estimated in hematoxylin and eosin (H&E) stained sections by the presence of a cluster of relatively clear staining cells within a lymphocytic focus. More specific identification of germinal centers requires immunohistochemical staining for follicular dendritic cells with anti-CD21 or CD23 [4, 9].

There is no standardization of labial salivary gland biopsies in SS, but there are several points of importance in LSGB. The first issue refers to a sufficient amount of glandular tissue. A reasonable compromise is four glands, although a minimum sized evaluable surface area (8 mm^2) may be achieved with 2–3 glands. The largest possible area to be sampled would give the best results, but a larger operative field increases the surgical risk. On the other hand, some glands may be atrophic or damaged, and the volume of the material obtained through the biopsy should be sufficient to overcome this artifact and achieve a valid result. It is more recommended to evaluate multiple different lobules than to concentrate on a single abnormal lobule, which may not be typical of the entire gland. In routine management, H&E staining is used in order to determine these structures. For clinical trials, additional staining with CD21 as well as CD20 and CD3 is required. CD21 is a marker of follicular dendritic cells. Germinal centers should be reported and pathologists are advised to use caution in order to avoid overestimating germinal centers by relying solely on CD21. Furthermore, the distribution of the inflammatory cells in the gland may be uneven. Considering this uneven distribution, a single tissue section may result in underdiagnosis. While increasing the number of sections has the potential to reduce this problem, the optimal number of sections has yet to be determined. Some research suggests taking labial salivary glands at different depths from the same incision. Focus score can change significantly at different tissue depths within the minor salivary glands. Multiple sections for LSGB increase the diagnostic value and are more representative than a single section [7, 10] (**Figure 3**).

5. Limitations of the assessment of focus score

- Differentiation of FLS with nonspecific chronic sialadenitis and sclerosing chronic sialadenitis

- Severe acinar atrophy, interstitial fibrosis, and increase in fat cells in biopsy specimens

- Age-related features in biopsy specimens (increased fibrosis, acinar atrophy, and adipose tissue
- Lack of the measurement of the infiltrate [7]

6. Other histopathological features of LSGB

There are also other histopathological features in the labial glands that are associated with SS and therefore might be indicative of this disease. Lymphoepithelial lesions (LELs) are striated ducts, which are infiltrated by lymphocytes with concurrent hyperplasia of the epithelial cells. They are found both in parotid and labial glands, and are more representative of parotid glands than labial glands.

Severity of the LELs can be classified into three stages: stage 1: a partial LEL (affecting <50% of the epithelium), stage 2: developed LELS (affecting 50–100% of the epithelium), and stage 3: occluded LELs (fully circumferentially affected epithelium without lumen).

Besides LELs, the salivary gland of SS patients also presents a relative decrease in IgA + plasma cells. Several studies showed that a relative decrease of <70% IgA + plasma cells was more sensitive and more disease specific than the FS. Both features can help assess the salivary gland biopsies for the diagnosis of SS, especially when the FS in the biopsy is <1 [7, 19–23].

7. Alternative types of salivary gland biopsies in SS

The main alternative types of salivary gland biopsies in SS are parotid gland biopsy and sublingual gland biopsy. Parotid gland biopsy allows the clinician to monitor the disease progression and to assess the effect of an intervention treatment in SS. Parotid tissue can be harvested easily, repeated biopsies from the same parotid gland are possible, and the histopathologic results can be compared with other diagnostic results derived from the same gland, such as secretory function, sialographic appearance, and ultrasonography. Furthermore, parotid biopsy is better in the identification of lymphomas. The main possible complications are facial nerve damage, Frey's syndrome, and development of sialoceles and salivary fistulae. A temporary change in sensation in the skin area of the incision is also a well-documented complication after parotid biopsy. Some patients might also develop preauricular hypothesis, although this is usually temporary. Furthermore, in SS, the salivary gland tissue is replaced by fatty tissue, and the risk of harvesting fatty tissue is thereby increased if done by inexperienced physicians. Parotid biopsy is particularly recommended in pediatric patients in whom SS is suspected and who have a negative minor salivary gland biopsy result. Incisional biopsy of the parotid gland overcomes most of the disadvantages of labial biopsy. When evaluating the parotid and labial biopsy, sensitivity and specificity are comparable, estimated to be 78 and 86%, respectively. Comparative studies suggest that both procedures—sublingual and parotid biopsy—retain a diagnostic potential comparable to that of lip biopsy and may be associated with lower postoperative morbidity. A comparison of sublingual gland biopsy with labial gland biopsy is better than that of labial gland biopsy, whereas the specificity of the latter is greater than that of the former. Sublingual gland biopsy is a relatively safe procedure, although the postoperative complications of sublingual salivary gland biopsy include ligaturing the Wharton duct, resulting from the placement of sutures, bleeding, and swelling in the floor of the mouth. Damage to the lingual nerve related to this biopsy technique has never been reported in the literature. No specialized histopathologic criteria have been established for the diagnosis of SS after a sublingual gland biopsy, and researchers merely used the criteria for labial gland biopsies [24–28].

8. Oral involvement and xerostomia

The rate of dry mouth in SS ranged from 41% at initial diagnosis to 84% 10 years after diagnosis. Hyposalivation or xerostomia measured by sialometry is one of the objective clinical criteria in the diagnosis of SS. According to the current classification criteria of SS, an unstimulated salivary flow rate of 0.1 ml/minute in sialometry gives a score of 1 to the weighted sum of 5 items. Dryness is also a subjective symptom of SS and is associated with many clinical implications. There are two possible sources of hyposalivation. The first possible origin is the presence of mononuclear cell aggregates around the ducts and acini of salivary glands resulting in functional and structural alterations of these glands and impairing their secretory function. In addition to the direct relationship between mononuclear cell infiltrations and secretory function, there are alternative pathways, such as induction of apoptosis of epithelial glands, alterations in aquaporin distribution, or inhibition of neurotransmission by antimuscarinic antibodies, lead to impaired glandular homeostasis. The second proposed hypothesis is the destruction of the duct and acinar cells of the salivary glands, and neural degeneration and/or the inhibition of nerve transmission. Hyposialia or decreased salivation can lead to xerostomia with clinical oral symptoms [29]. Dry mouth is associated with both objective and subjective signs and symptoms. The most common complaints related to dry mouth are presented in **Table 3**.

In SS, the gingiva and mucosa of the oral cavity are not protected by salivary mucins, leading to less lubrication of the tissues. This can cause signs such as oral mucosal inflammation, mucosal sloughing, erythematous mucosa, and traumatic ulcers. Patients may demonstrate depapillation of the tongue in advanced cases. With time, the concentration of lactoferrin, potassium and cystatin C in saliva grows, while the amylase and carbonic anhydrase concentration drops. Decreased secretion of saliva, the loss of its buffer properties, and a lower concentration of saliva proteins such as histatins, mucins, IgA, and proteins rich in proline and statherins increase the risk of opportunistic infections, mainly fungal infections by *Candida albicans*. The prevalence of *Candida albicans* is >68% in patients with SS. Oral candidiasis may be asymptomatic or may show as fissured tongue, rhomboid mid-tongue, nonspecific ulcerations, prosthetic stomatopathies, or generalized candidiasis. It most often takes the form of chronic candidiasis, and less often of pseudodiphtheritic candidiasis. Candida infections often present as atrophic or erythematous candidiasis and are associated with a burning mouth, which is described by approximately one-third of patients with SS. In SS patients,

A dryness of the mouth in the morning and at night
A frequent need to sip water
A lip dryness, exfoliation, fissuring
A predisposition to aphthae, ulcers, and mouth sores
A burning sensation in the mouth
A dysphagia
A dysgeusia

Table 3.
The most common complaints related to dry mouth.

Candidiasis
Angular cheilitis
Simple cheilitis
Exfoliative cheilitis
Aphthae
Aphthoid lesions
Nonspecific ulcerations
Paleness of the oral mucosa
Staphylococcal infection

Table 4.
Symptoms of oral mucosa in the Sjögren's syndrome.

C. albicans, *C. tropicalis*, *C. glabrata*, and *C. parapsilosis* are mainly isolated. Apart from oral candidiasis, a number of other changes and symptoms regarding the oral mucosa may occur (**Table 4**).

Angular cheilitis may be accompanied with fungal infection. In simple cheilitis, dominant manifestations are lip exfoliation and cracking, their proneness to bleeding, periodic swelling, and burning. The lesions are mostly limited to lip vermillion, less often labial mucosa or the facial skin around the vermillion is affected. In exfoliative cheilitis, thick brown keratin plaques are also formed. Skin redness over the lip vermillion and swelling are more often observed [29].

SS patients are predisposed to rampant caries and traumatic oral lesions. Lack of antibacterial salivary proteins results in severe tooth caries, especially on the unexposed tooth spaces. Rampant cervical caries is the most typical manifestation to SS.

9. Laryngological and otological manifestations of SS

The lymphocytic infiltrations are representative for all salivary glands and have other possible consequences. Although the sicca syndrome prevails, in a clinical presentation, a bilateral parotid swelling induced by progressive lymphocyte infiltration leads both to ductal inflammation and acinar destruction in about 50% of patients. Recurrent swelling and inflammations of the parotid or submandibular glands in SS are well documented. Slow salivary flow, acinar destruction, and lymphocytic infiltrations predispose to inflammation and salivary gland enlargement. This enlargement should be distinguished from lymphomas. The most significant complication of SS is the development of lymphoproliferative malignancy, which occurs in about 5% of SS patients. Malignant lymphoma, particularly mucosa-associated lymphoid tissue (MALT) lymphoma, is relatively a frequent complication of SS with an incidence ranging between 5 and 10% and a median time from SS to lymphoma diagnosis of 7.5 years. Lymphomas accompanying SS can be confirmed by histopathological examination of salivary gland biopsy. The detection of germinal centers (GC) in salivary gland biopsy can be a very sensitive and predictive feature for lymphogenesis. Antigen-driven B cell selection normally takes place in GC within secondary lymphoid organs, but there is conclusive evidence that also ectopic GC in the salivary glands of SS patients allow affinity maturation of GC B cells with somatic Ig gene hypermaturation. Parotid gland biopsy is more recommended for diagnosis of lymphomas than labial salivary glands [7, 18–23].

Dryness of the mucosa of the upper respiratory tract is a predominant symptom and results in nasal, oropharynx, nasopharynx, laryngopharynx, vocal cord dryness, and dryness of the skin of the external auditory meatus. The main laryngological symptoms accompanying SS include the following:

- Dry nose with congestion, crusting, and epistaxis
- Dryness, crusting, or atrophy of the nasal mucosa
- Soreness and/or dryness of the throat
- Viscid secretions on the posterior pharyngeal wall and tenacious mucus over the vocal cords
- Dry wax and a "milky" appearance of the tympanic membrane
- Dysphagia
- Hoarseness
- Otalgia
- Tinnitus
- A chronic dry cough
- Dyspnea
- Gastrotracheal reflux
- Otitis externa
- Myringitis
- Sensorineural hearing loss
- Facial hypaesthesia and trigeminal nerve neuropathy, and multiple cranial neuropathy [30–33]

Other possible laryngological manifestations of SS are early and progressive hearing loss and symptoms related to neuropathy of the eighth cranial nerve. Approximately, a quarter of patients suffer from high-frequency hearing loss of cochlear origin, as detected by impedance audiometry or auditory brainstem procedures. The immunologic theory of sensorineural hearing loss (SNHL) in SS is based on antibody activity and cytotoxic T-cell-mediated apoptosis in the inner ear. It has been suggested that these autoantibodies induce thrombosis in the labyrinthine vessels, thereby causing damage to the inner ear, resulting in SNHL. The majority of primary SS patients exhibit hearing impairments of cochlear origin, principally at high frequencies. Sensorineural damage may be attributable to vasculitis or neuritis, or may represent an ototoxic effect of the drugs used to treat primary SS. Although there is no evidence of damage to the central auditory pathways in SS, these patients tend to have a higher prevalence of sensorineural hearing impairment compared with the general population. Idiopathic hearing loss may represent the initial manifestation of systemic vasculitis, including SS. The pathomechanisms underlying cranial neuropathy in SS have not yet been explained, except for trigeminal neuropathy due to ganglionopathy. The two possible mechanisms, vascular origin with damage to the vasa nervorum, and an immunologic cause inducing lymphocytic infiltration of the nerve have been suggested in nerve palsies related to SS. Vasculitis in peripheral neuropathy and ganglionopathy in trigeminal or ataxic neuropathies have been reported as the main pathogenic etiology. The rapid and almost complete recovery from nerve palsy after therapy with corticosteroids and azathioprine suggests that lymphocytic infiltrate, rather than a vasculitic process, was the cause of cranial neuropathy in SS [33–40].

Author details

Bartłomiej Kamiński[1]* and Katarzyna Błochowiak[2]

1 Department of Otolaryngology, District Hospital, Skarzysko-Kamienna, Poland

2 Department of Oral Surgery, Poznan University of Medical Sciences, Poznan, Poland

*Address all correspondence to: bartl.kaminski@gmail.com

References

[1] Shiboski CH, Shiboski SC, Seror R. 2016 America College of Rheumatology/ European League Against Rheumatism Classification Criteria for primary Sjögren's syndrome. Arthritis & Rhematology. 2017;**69**:35-45

[2] Shiboski CH, Shiboski SC, le Seror R, Criswell LA, Labetoulle M, Lietman TM, et al. American College of Rheumatology/ European League Against Rheumatism Classification Criteria for Primary Sjögren's Syndrome. A consensus and data-driven methodology involving three international patient cohorts. Annals of the Rheumatic Diseases. 2017;**76**:9-16

[3] Mavragani CP, Moutsopoulos HM. Sjögren's syndrome. Annual Review of Pathology: Mechanisms of Disease. 2014;**9**:273-285

[4] Daniels TE, Cox D, Shiboski CH, Schiødt M, Wu A, Lanfranchi H, et al. Greenspan JS and for the Sjögren's international collaborative clinical Alliance (SICCA) research groups. Associations between salivary gland histopathologic diagnoses and phenotypic features of Sjögren's syndrome (SS) among 1726 registry participants. Arthritis and Rheumatism. 2011;**63**:2021-2030

[5] Pereira DL, Vilela VS, Dos Santos TC, Pires FR. Clinical and laboratorial profile and histological features on minor salivary glands from patients under investigation for Sjögren's syndrome. Medicina Oral, Patología Oral y Cirugía Bucal. 2014;**19**:e237-e241

[6] Kim J, Sun D, Ozl R, Graderbeck T, Birnbaum J, Akpek EK, et al. A validated method of labial minor salivary gland biopsy for the diagnosis of Sjögren's syndrome. The Laryngoscope. 2016;**126**:2041-2046

[7] Kroese F, Haacke E, Bombardieri M. The role of salivary gland histopathology in primary Sjögren's syndrome: Promises and pitfalls. Clinical and Experimental Rheumatology. 2018;**36**(Suppl 112): 222-233

[8] Delli K, Vissink A, Spijkervet FKL. Salivary gland biopsy for Sjögren's syndrome. Oral and Maxillofacial Surgery Clinics of North America. 2014;**26**(1):23-33

[9] Franceschini F, Cavazzana I, Andreoli L, Tincani A. The 2016 classification criteria for primary Sjogren's syndrome: What's new? BMC Medicine. 2017;**15**:69

[10] Sarioğlu S, Küçük Ŭ, Cetin P, Sari I, Bĭrlĭk AM. Minor salivary gland evaluation: Sjögren's syndrome. Turk J Med Sci. 2016;**46**:63-65

[11] Varela-Centelles P, Sanchez-Sanchez M, Seoane J. Lip biopsy for the diagnosis of Sjögren's syndrome: Beware of the punch. International Journal of Oral and Maxillofacial Surgery. 2014;**43**(1):127-130

[12] Giovelli RA, Santos MCS, Serrano E, Valim V. Clinical characteristics and biopsy accuracy in suspected cases of Sjögren's syndrome referred to labial salivary gland biopsy. BMC Musculoskeletal Disorders. 2015;**16**:30

[13] Bamba R, Sweiss NJ, Langerman AJ, Taxy JB, Blair EA. The minor salivary gland biopsy as a diagnostic tool for Sjögren's syndrome. The Laryngoscope. 2009;**119**:1922-1926

[14] Langerman AJ, Blair EA, Sweiss NJ, Taxy JB. Utility of lip biopsy in the diagnosis and treatment of Sjögren's syndrome. The Laryngoscope. 2007;**117**(6):1004-1008

[15] Van Stein-Callenfels D, Tan J, Bloemena E, van Vugt RM, Voskuyl

AE, Santana NT, et al. The role of labial salivary gland biopsy in the diagnostic procedure for Sjögren's syndrome; a study of 94 cases. Medicina Oral, Patología Oral y Cirugía Bucal. 2014;**19**(4):e372-e376

[16] Tarpley TM Jr, Anderson LG, White CL. Minor salivary gland involvement in Sjögren's syndrome. Oral Surgery, Oral Medicine, and Oral Pathology. 1974;**37**(1):64-74

[17] Chisholm DM, Mason DK. Labial salivary gland biopsy in Sjögren's disease. Journal of Clinical Pathology. 1968;**21**(5):656-660

[18] Keszler A, Adler LI, Gandolfo MS, Masquijo Bisio PA, Smith AC, Vollenweider CF, et al. MALT lymphoma in labial salivary gland biopsy from Sjögren syndrome: Importance of follow-up in early detection. Oral Surgery, Oral Medicine, Oral Pathology, Oral Radiology. 2013;**115**:e28-e33

[19] Theander E, Vasaitis L, Baecklund E, Nordmark G, Warfvinge G, Liedholm R, et al. Lymphoid organisation in labial salivary gland biopsies is a possible predictor for the development of malignant lymphoma in primary Sjögren's syndrome. Annals of the Rheumatic Diseases. 2011;**70**:1363-1368

[20] Bende RJ, Slot LM, Hoogeboom R, Wormhoudt TA, Adeoye AO, Guikema JE, et al. Stereotypic rheumatoid factors that are frequently expressed in mucosa-associated lymphoid tissue-type lymphomas are rare in the labial salivary glands of patients with Sjögren's syndrome. Arthritis & Rhematology. 2015;**67**:1074-1083

[21] Ferro F, Marcucci E, Orlandi M, Baldini C, Bartoloni-Bocci E. One year in review 2017: Primary Sjögren's syndrome. Clinical and Experimental Rheumatology. 2017;**35**:179-191

[22] Fragoulis GE, Fragkioudaki S, Reilly JH, Kerr SC, McInnes IB, Mautsopoulos HM. Analysis of the cell populations composing the mononuclear cell infiltrates in the labial minor salivary glands from patients with rheumatoid arthritis and sicca syndrome. Journal of Autoimmunity. 2016;**73**:85-91

[23] Soyfoo MS, Catteau X, Delporte C. Parotid gland biopsy as an additional diagnostic tool for supporting the diagnosis of Sjögren's syndrome. International Journal of Rheumatology. 2011:302527

[24] Pijpe J, Kalk WWI, van der Wal JE, et al. Parotid gland biopsy compared with labial biopsy in the diagnosis of patients with primary Sjögren's syndrome. Rheumatology. 2007;**46**(10):335-341

[25] de Sousa Gomes P, Juodzbalys G, Fernandes MH, Guobis Z. Diagnostic approaches to Sjögren's syndrome: A literature review and own clinical experience. Journal of Oral & Maxillofacial Research. 2012;**3**(1):e3

[26] Błochowiak K, Wyganowska-Świątkowska M. Labial minor salivary gland biopsy in the diagnosis of Sjögren syndrome-own experience. Dent Forum. 2018;**46**(2):17-21

[27] Scardina GA, Spanó G, Carini F, et al. Diagnostic evaluation of serial sections of labial salivary gland biopsies in Sjögren's syndrome. Medicina Oral, Patología Oral y Cirugía Bucal. 2007;**12**:565-568

[28] Błochowiak K, Olewicz-Gawlik A, Polańska A, Nowak-Gabryel M, Kocięcki J, Witmanowski H, et al. Oral mucosal manifestations in primary and secondary Sjögren syndrome and dry mouth syndrome. Postępy Dermatologii i Alergologii. 2016;**33**:23-27

[29] Öztürk AB, Öztürk E, Kasapoğlu E. Chronic cough due to mucosal dryness

in primary Sjögren's syndrome: A case report. Tüberküloz ve Toraks. 2014;**62**:243-244

[30] Kumon Y, Kakigi A, Sugiura T. Clinical images: Otalgia, an unusual complication of Sjögren's syndrome. Arthritis and Rheumatism. 2009;**60**:2542

[31] Fox RI. Sjögren's syndrome. Lancet. 2005;**366**:321-331

[32] Calzada AP, Balaker AE, Ishiyama G, Lopez IA, Ishiyama A. Temporal bone histopathology and immunoglobulin deposition in Sjogren's syndrome. Otology & Neurotology. 2012;**33**:258-266

[33] Kamiński B. Laryngological manifestations of Sjögren's syndrome. Reumatologia/Rheumatology. 2019;**57**(1):37-44

[34] Kim KS, Kim HS. Successful treatment of sensorineural hearing loss in Sjögren's syndrome with corticosteroid. The Korean Journal of Internal Medicine. 2016;**31**:612-615

[35] Ramos-Casals M, Tzioufas AG, Font J. Primary Sjögren's syndrome: New clinical and therapeutic concepts. Annals of the Rheumatic Diseases. 2005;**64**:347-354

[36] Hadithi M, Stam F, Donker AJ, Dijkmans BA. Sjögren's syndrome: An unusual cause of Bell's palsy. Annals of the Rheumatic Diseases. 2001;**60**:724-725

[37] Ashraf VV, Bhasi R, Kumar RP, Girija AS. Primary Sjögren's syndrome manifesting as multiple cranial neuropathies: MRI findings. Annals of Indian Academy of Neurology. 2009;**12**:124-126

[38] Sakai K, Hamaguchi T, Yamada M. Multiple cranial nerve enhancement on MRI in primary Sjögren's syndrome. Internal Medicine. 2010;**49**:857-859

[39] Tucci M, Quatraro C, Silvestris F. Sjögren's syndrome: An autoimmune disorder with otolaryngological involvement. Acta Otorhinolaryngologica Italica. 2005;**25**:139-144

[40] Birnbaum J. Facial Weakness, Otalgia, and Hemifacial Spasm: A Novel Neurological Syndrome in a Case-Series of 3 Patient

Section 2

IgG4 Related Diseases

Chapter 5

IgG4-Related Disease and the Spectrum of Mimics in Rheumatology

Agata Sebastian, Piotr Donizy and Piotr Wiland

Abstract

Immunoglobulin G4 (IgG4)-related disease (IgG4-RD) is an immune-mediated condition that can affect almost any organ. It is a chronic, systemic, inflammatory condition of unknown etiology. Pseudotumor formation is the most common and characteristic clinical symptom. The variable organ dysfunction reflects the clinical presentation. Because there are not specific antibodies for this disease, histopathological assessment provide the pivotal role in the diagnosis. IgG4-RD is characterized by a lymphoplasmacytic infiltrate composed of IgG4+ plasma cells, storiform fibrosis, obliterative phlebitis and mild to moderate eosinophilia. In this chapter we present the newest knowledge of the IgG4-RD pathogenesis and then concentrate on clinical symptoms which can mimic many other conditions in rheumatology, e.g., this common as Sjögren syndrome or rare as vasculitis or idiopathic retroperitoneal fibrosis.

Keywords: IgG4-related disease, Mikulicz syndrome, Kuttner's disease, pseudotumor

1. Spectrum of IgG4-related disease

IgG4-related disease (IgG4-RD) belongs to quite new disease entities; its name was introduced in the 21st century. In the course of the disease, characteristic infiltrates are formed, composed of mononuclear cells, mainly IgG4 cells. Also, fibrosis of affected organs is observed. In the majority of patients, concomitant increase in serum IgG4 concentration is found, but not in every patient [1, 2].

Location of lesions	Name of IgG-RD disease
- pancreas	- Autoimmune pancreatitis type 1, AIP
- biliary ducts	- IgG4-related sclerosing cholangitis
- parotid glands, submandibular glands and lacrimal glands	- IgG4-related sialadenitis, IgG4-related dacryoadenitis
-lacrimal glands and oculomotor muscles and orbit	- IgG4-related pan-orbital inflammation, IgG4-related orbital pseudotumor
- retroperitoneal space	- IgG4-related retroperitoneal fibrosis
-aorta	- IgG4-related aortitis/periaortitis
- kidneys	- IgG4-related kidney disease
- lungs	- IgG4-related lung disease
- lymph nodes	- IgG4-related lymphadenopathy

Table 1.
Current nomenclature of most common clinical forms of IgG4-RD.

In 2011, classification criteria were presented with a spectrum of diseases described so far in medicine that may correspond to IgG4-RD. The first relationship between autoimmune pancreatitis and increased serum IgG4 was observed in 2001 and it is one of the most common manifestations of IgG4-RD-type 1 of autoimmune pancreatitis [3]. Currently, there is a tendency to introduce the name IgG4-RD disease depending on the location of the lesions (**Table 1**) [4].

Due to possible location of pathologic lesions in most of the organs, every physician may have contact with IgG4-RD, independent of his/her speciality.

2. Epidemiology

The disease develops mostly in men, middle-aged or older. The ratio of disease incidence in men vs. women is between 1:0.77 and 4:1 [5, 6]. The disease incidence is not fully known and it seems that it varies significantly for different parts of the world. The highest number of IgG4-RD cases has been reported so far for Asia. In Japan, based on the register of patients with IgG4-RD, the disease incidence was determined to be 0.28–1.08 in 100,000 people [7]. Despite the fact that the disease is not often seen in children, there were more than a dozen such cases reported in the world [8]. In the case of an affected aorta, lesions in the course of IgG4-RD were observed in 4–20% of patients, depending on a publication [9–11].

3. Pathogenesis of IgG4-RD

Pathogenesis of IgG4-RD is not fully understood. It seems that many factors contribute to disease development, including allergic, autoimmune and genetic factors [12].

The observed positive response to drugs blocking B-lymphocyte activity and monoclonal increase of IgG4 concentration suggested a significant role of B lymphocytes in the initiation and maintenance of the disease process [13]. However, current research indicates inappropriate activation of T lymphocytes causing autoimmune defect.

The first publications indicated an increase of Th2 cytokine production in patients with IgG4-RD [14, 15]. However, it turned out that this effect is seen only in patients with IgG4-RD and concomitant allergic symptoms [16]. It was shown that in response to Th2-dependent cytokines, such as interleukin 4, 5, 10, and 13, as well as transforming growth factor beta (TGF-β), the eosinophil number and concentration of IgG4 and IgE increase and fibrosis progresses [17]. Eosinophilia, similarly to allergy, may occur in 1/3 of patients with IgG4-RD. However, the correlation between the increased number of eosinophils and clinical symptoms of allergy was not confirmed. Similarly, allergic symptoms did not correlate in patients with IgG4-RD with increased IgE concentration [18]. Allergic symptoms included allergic rhinitis, nasal polyps, bronchial asthma and atopic dermatitis [19]. Further studies showed that a key role in the pathomechanism of IgG4-RD play T follicular helper cells (Tfh) and regulatory T cells (Treg). Their role is particularly seen in relation with class switching of B cells and induction of aberrant lymphoid follicle formation in tissue. However, Il-21 and Il-4 related to Tfh play a great role in the formation of germinal centers, differentiation of B lymphocytes, induction of plasmoblasts and the phenomenon of class switching leading to the production of igG4 [20, 21]. This is in the Tfh germinal centers of lymph nodes that Il-4 is produced and long-lasting memory lymphocytes responsible for disease recurrences proliferate [22, 23].

The analyses of immunophenotyping of Thf subclasses showed that in IgG4-RD, cytokines type Th2 (IL-4, IL-5, IL-13) are produced by cells not expressing CXCR3 and CCR6 [24]. The number of Th2 cells is increased in IgG4 and correlates with increased IgG4 concentration in serum and IL4, the number of plasmocytes and the number of affected organs [21, 25]. However, in AIP, an increased number of CD4+ and CD25+ Treg was observed [21, 25]. In the most recent reports, attention has been paid to cytotoxic lymphocytes CD4+ (CTLs) [26–29] as well as the possibility of participation of annexin A11 in the pathogenesis of AIP [30].

The role of plasmoblasts and IgG4 itself is still not known in the pathomechanism of IgG4-RD. It is thought that they are more of disease markers than factors of disease development [5, 22]. Among IgG, there are 4 subclasses in humans (IgG1-IgG4). Normally, IgG4 constitute about 2–3% of all IgG, and their serum concentration is 35–51 mg/dL on average. Higher serum concentration of IgG4 was observed in men and in the elderly [31]. IgG4 and IgE are usually produced as a result of chronic exposure to antigens [32] or after allergy immunotherapy [33]. IgG4 is not able to form immunocomplexes which could stimulate antigen-presenting cells and enhance immunological response. Moreover, it does not initiate the classic pathway of complement activation [34]. The IgG4 antibodies bind weakly to complement C1q and Fcγ receptors. As a consequence, they are not involved in antibody-dependent cell-mediated cytotoxicity [35]. Additionally, IgG4 antibodies are dynamic molecules—altering their properties by spontaneous exchange of one of the two Fab fragments between individual immunoglobulin molecules. This process involves dissociation of immunoglobulin G4 heavy-chain dimers and a subsequent bonding of each IgG4 half-molecule with a different IgG4 half-molecule. This half-molecule exchange yields bi-specific antibodies able to bind with two different antigens, but monovalent for each of them. These properties of IgG4 molecules are the reason why IgG4 antibodies do not bind to the complement directly, do not initiate the classic pathway of complement activation, or why they are poor Fc receptor activators. This reduced IgG4 effector function has been responsible for these antibodies being considered anti-inflammatory [31]. IgG4 are believed to constitute a veritable antigen "garbage disposal" system, which can attenuate inflammation or protect against type I hypersensitivity by inhibiting IgE activity, as well as prevent type II and III hypersensitivity by blocking immune complex formation [36, 37].

Genetic studies seem to confirm some genetic background of IgG4-RD. Until present, differences in the expression of different genes have been found in salivary glands of patients with Sjögren syndrome and in patients with IgG4-RD, compared to healthy population. Only in a group of patients with IgG4-RD, overexpression of genes related to cell proliferation, organization of extracellular matrix and tissue fibrosis was confirmed [38]. Also, the relationship was found between AIP and class II antigen of the major histocompatibility complex HLA-DRB1*0405-DQB1*0401 and nuclear factor κB gene polymorphism and a molecule for type Fc-3 receptor on B cells [39].

4. Clinical manifestations of IgG4-RD

In the course of IgG4-RD, infiltrations composed mainly of IgG4 are formed, and characteristic fibrosis of affected organs is seen. These lesions usually form pseudotumors, which may occur in every organ. Most commonly observed locations of IgG4-RD are shown in **Table 2**. Single clinical cases of disease occurrence in the brain and cerebrospinal meninges, as well as intestines, causing ileus, have also been reported [40, 41]. IgG4-RD may affect one organ or occur in a generalized form. It seems that some locations may be more common for a particular sex. For example, lesions in the pancreas are more common in men, while sialadenitis

1. Characteristic symptoms of organ affection with its enlargement, or abnormal function of organ/organs 2. Increased serum IgG4 concentration ≥ 135 mg/dL 3. Characteristic changes in histopathological examination: • infiltration composed of lymphocytes and plasmatic cells and fibrosis • infiltration of IgG4+ cells: >10 cells IgG4+ hpf in a high-resolution microscope and quantitative ratio of IgG4+/IgG > 40%
Certain diagnosis of IgG4-RD: meeting the requirements of 1, 2, 3 Probable diagnosis of IgG4-R: meeting the requirements of 1 and 3 Possible diagnosis of IgG4-RD: meeting the requirement of 1 and 2

Table 2.
Criteria of IgG4-RD diagnosis.

and dacryoadenitis in women [42]. Patients with IgG4-usually do not present general symptoms such as fever, night sweats, or weight loss [43].

5. Criteria of IgG4-RD diagnosis

Criteria of IgG4-RD diagnosis were developed in 2012 (**Table 2**) [44].

Summing up the criteria of IgG4-RD diagnosis: one of the most important examinations in case of an appropriate clinical picture of the disease is the histopathological examination of the affected organ. It is now believed to be the key examination. In the next chapter, the principles of histopathological examination are presented, depending on the location of the pathological lesions.

In the second point of the criteria, IgG4 serum concentration was also included. It should be minimum 135 mg/dL in an affected individual. The probability of IgG4-RD diagnosis is significantly increased when this concentration is higher than 270 mg/dL [45]. However, it should be remembered that in some patients with IgG4-RD, an increase of serum IgG4 is observed. This percentage may be as high as 40% [46, 47]. IgG4 production depends mainly on the action of interleukin 6 and 10. Moreover, it was observed that in some autoimmune diseases, the concentration of IgG4 is also increased. Among others, in primary Sjögren syndrome, in systemic lupus erythematosus, and rheumatoid arthritis. A similar situation was also observed in 2% of patients with cancers and in healthy population [46, 47].

In IgG4-RD, no other immunologic markers observed in rheumatoid diseases are found, including antinuclear antibodies, ANCA antibodies or decreased complement components C3 and C4 [48].

In 1/3 of patients, eosinophilia in the peripheral blood is observed [18]. However, it does not correlate with the allergic symptoms [19].

In the diagnostics of IgG4-RD, imaging plays an important role, depending on lesion location, e.g., PET, magnetic resonance, computed tomography, EUS, bronchoscopy. However, the disease has no sufficiently characteristic image in any of the imaging methods, therefore these examinations are helpful in the evaluation of the affected organs and selection of the biopsy site, but they cannot be the only methods of disease diagnosis.

Another most important component of the criteria is their application only after exclusion of all other diseases that may suggest IgG4-RD disease, including cancer. It was evaluated that neoplastic lesions may occur even in 7% of patients with IgG4-RD. Development of neoplastic lesions, including lymphomas, was reported even after 5 years from diagnosis of IgG4-RD in the orbit, with affected salivary glands and cerebrospinal meninges [49, 50]. On the other hand, there are publications denying the increased risk of cancer development in IgG4-RD [51, 52].

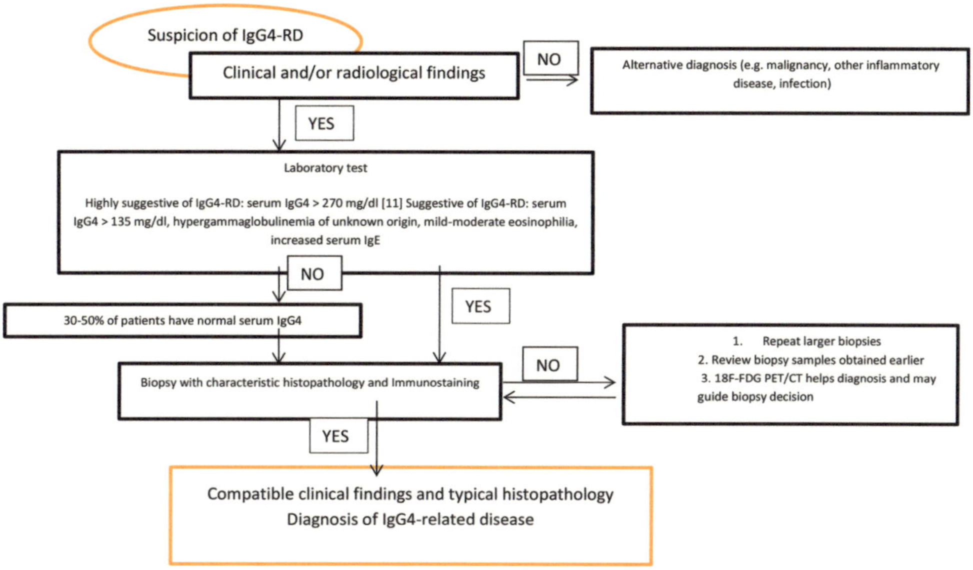

Figure 1.
Diagnostic scheme in IgG4-RD [22, 37, 54].

An interesting fact is that most cancers observed in patients with IgG4-RD do not contain IgG4 cells [5]. At present, there are no well-designed observational studies confirming these findings. Therefore, patients with lesions in the clinical picture or patients not responding to basic treatment, should have their diagnosis verified.

The diagnostics of lesions within large salivary and lacrimal glands should take the primary Sjögren syndrome into consideration. One of the key clinical differences is the lack of symptoms of dryness confirmed in objective examinations in patients with IgG4-RD [47, 53] and the lack of immunological markers characteristic for the Sjögren syndrome.

Taking the above into consideration, diagnostic and therapeutic procedures were developed in 2015 in patients with suspected IgG4-RD, which is presented in **Figure 1** [22, 54].

New classification guidelines were presented, during the ACR meeting in Chicago in October 2018. It were developed by 79 experts from five continents and are awaiting approval by ACR and the EULAR. The guidelines based on clinical findings, bloodwork, radiologic findings and exclusion criteria for other mimickers.

6. Organ location of lesions in IgG4-RD

The lesions may occur individually or in many organs at the same time. From the point of view of rheumatologists, the most important locations include the below mentioned organs.

6.1 IgG4-RD of the head and neck

Lesions located within the head and neck belong to the most common clinical manifestation of IgG4-RD [55, 56]. They can affect large salivary glands (submandibular salivary glands, parotid glands), thyroid, lacrimal glands, orbit with oculomotor muscles, nasal sinuses, and upper airways. Mikulicz's disease is an enlargement (usually symmetrical) of lacrimal glands, parotid and submandibular glands, and sometimes sublingual glands. In the past, Mikulicz's disease was believed to be a subtype of Sjögren syndrome. Today we know that these are two different disease entities with a different treatment response. Diagnostic criteria of Mikulicz's disease include: symmetric oedema of at least two pairs of lacrimal glands, parotid or submandibular glands, present for at least 3 months, and increased serum concentration, of IgG4 > 135 mg/dL, as well as a typical histopathological picture of the affected tissues.

The term Kuttner's tumor is used in case of submandibular salivary gland enlargement.

In case of lesions located in the orbit, vision disturbances, orbital pain, swelling of the eyelids caused by infiltration of oculomotor muscles and infiltration of tumor mass in the orbit may occur. Sometimes these changes may occur in tissues around the orbit as painless facial swelling. Cases of IgG4-RD were reported with infiltration and destruction of bone tissues, resulting in a saddle-shaped nose [57]. The basis for diagnosis is always a histopathological examination.

Involvement of the thyroid in IgG4-RD is possible. Recently, a lot of effort was put into this issue. First, based on case reports, it was found that Riedel thyroiditis belongs to IgG4 diseases. Some authors suggest also that the form of Hashimoto's thyroiditis with fibrosis, leading to hypothyroidism is also caused by IgG4-RD. This could be indicated by more common occurrence of hypothyroidism in patients with autoimmune pancreatitis and IgG4-RD [58–60].

6.2 Location in the lungs, mediastinum and pleura

Lesions located in the lungs may occur in the form of pseudotumors, "milk glass" lesions, lesions resembling interstitial lung disease or honeycomb lung. Less commonly, thickening of bronchovascular bundles and interlobular septa may occur. Also, involvement of the pleura and mediastinum was reported—infiltration with lymph node enlargement. In case of disease diagnosis in this location, biopsy with a thorough differential diagnosis is needed, including cancer, vasculitis [61–63].

6.3 IgG4-RD in the alimentary tract

The first organ in which IgG4-RD was reported was pancreas. Autoimmune symptoms of pancreatitis type I include jaundice, abdominal pain, pruritus, de novo diabetes and fatty diarrhea [64–67].

Lesions characteristic for IgG4-RD may be also located in other parts of the alimentary tract, e.g., gallbladder or intestines. Clinical symptoms depend on the location of lesions and organ dysfunction caused by infiltration. They may be symptomless, as in the case of IgG4-RD findings in the removed gallbladders, or present as full-blown intestinal obstruction [47]. Involvement of bile ducts is well documented in the literature as IgG4-RD sclerosing cholangitis [68].

6.4 Lesions in the kidneys

Most commonly, tubulointerstitial inflammation is found in the course of IgG4-RD (IgG4-TIN) [69]. Rarely tumor masses in the kidneys or damage to the glomeruli are observed. However, such locations of IgG4-RD may be found in the literature too [70]. Moreover, involvement of the kidneys may be divided into directly related to the location of infiltration in the parenchyma, and indirectly related to infiltration of structures of the urinary system in the course of retroperitoneal fibrosis. Recently, also a case of renal amyloidosis AA in the course of IgG4-RD was reported. It is estimated that kidney involvement occurs in about 15% patients with IgG4-RD [70]. Besides symptoms of renal insufficiency in patients with IgG4-TIN, increased serum concentration of IgG and IgG4 is observed. In 60% of patients also hypocomplementemia is observed, in 40% eosinophilia and even in 32% antinuclear antibodies [71, 72]. In the imaging examinations, lesions in the course of IgG4-RD had a form of numerous hypodense lesions [69, 73]. At present, in diagnostics of renal lesions typical for IgG4-RD, criteria proposed by Mayo Clinic or criteria of the Japanese Society of Nephrology may be used [69, 74]. Their use does not require unconditional kidney biopsy. Considering the fact that lesions in the course of IgG4-RD are most commonly located also in other organs, biopsy of other organs is acceptable.

The most common histopathological form of IgG4-RD in the kidneys is membranous nephropathy (IgG4-MGN). Lesions in the glomeruli may be isolated or occur together with TIN, which is seen more often. The infiltrate observed in IgG4-MGN composed of IgG4 cells in the wall of glomerular capillaries may imitate primary membranous nephritis. Detection of antibodies against phospholipase A2 receptor (anti-PLA2R), which do not occur in IgG4-MGN, may be then helpful [70].

6.5 Involvement of the vessels in IgG4-RD

Lesions of IgG4-RD type usually locate in the aorta in the form of periaortitis, aortic dilatation, and aneurysm. The lesions are usually found in the abdominal aorta [9]. Inflammatory aortic aneurysm is characterized by thickening of the aortic wall, partial fibrosis of adventitia and infiltration composed of inflammatory cells [75]. Similar changes without enlargement of vessel diameter are called periaortitis [9]. The most characteristic location of inflammatory infiltrations for IgG4-RD is the adventitia (external fibrous membrane). In case of thoracic aorta involvement, separation of the aortic layers, lymphoplasmacytic aortitis and isolated aortitis are observed [76, 77]. Arterial wall thickening is relatively low compared to lesions found in the abdominal section. In some patients, aorta involvement may occur as unexpected separation of the aortic layers or sudden cardiac death; other changes in the course of the disease were rarely reported in vessels such as carotid artery, coronary arteries, pulmonary arteries, visceral vessels, mesentery vessels, iliac and vertebral arteries, brain vessels. If present, they were reported as vasculitis or aneurysms [78, 79].

The relationship between IgG4-RD and ANCA-associated vasculitis (AAV) has not been fully explained. It is known that these diseases have a similar clinical picture (asthma symptoms, involvement of nasal sinuses, involvement of lungs and kidneys) and may proceed with increased serum IgG4 concentration and eosinophilia in the peripheral blood. Most publications were dedicated to eosinophilic granulomatosis with vasculitis (EGPA) [9].

6.6 Location of IgG4-RD in the nervous system

Lesions in the central nervous system are rare. If present, they are usually found in the meninges of the brain or cranial nerves. The symptoms concerning cranial nerve involvement are most commonly caused by the presence of pseudotumors and pressure on or infiltration of the nerves [80].

6.7 Skin lesions in IgG4-RD

Skin lesions in the course of IgG4-RD are rarely observed and occur mainly in systemic forms. So far, the following skin lesions in the course of IgG4-RD were reported on: erythematous papules, tarsus and brown papules resembling nodular prurigo [81, 82].

6.8 Retroperitoneal fibrosis and IgG4-RD

Retroperitoneal fibrosis was reported in 13% of patients with multi-organ involvement in the course of IgG4-RD. Most of the lesions were periaortic or located around iliac vessels. In 33% of patients, hydronephrosis was found, more commonly of one kidney than two [83]. Classifying all cases of IgG4-RD as Ormond's disease is controversial if not confirmed by histopathology, and requires a further well-designed medical analysis. However such a suggestion was made in one publication [84].

6.9 Summary of the clinical picture

IgG4-RD is a disease of multiple systems. It may be located in one or in many organs at the same time. In case of suspected IgG4-RD, all other diseases which may mimic IgG4-RD should be excluded. For rheumatologists it is important to exclude in the differential diagnosis the following: neoplasms including solid lesions and lymphomas, inflammatory and infectious changes, sarcoidosis, vasculitis including granulomatous vasculitis, Sjögren syndrome, Castleman's disease, eosinophilic angiocentric fibrosis. As IgG4-RD may involve many organs, imaging diagnostics should always be carried out in order to determine all locations of the disease after diagnosis of the disease.

7. Histopathological evaluation in IgG4-RD

Histopathological evaluation is a crucial element of an accurate diagnosis of IgG4-RD due to their nonspecific clinical and laboratory features. Irrespective of the anatomic site, histopathologic presentation is similar and consists of five main histomorphological and immunohistochemical parameters evaluated in the tissue specimen (both biopsy and postoperative specimens) [1, 85, 86]:

1. dense lymphoplasmacytic infiltrate,

2. fibrosis with prominent storiform pattern,

3. obliterative phlebitis,

4. increased number of IgG4+ plasma cells/HPF - different cutoffs depending on the anatomic site and the type of evaluated material (biopsy vs. postoperative specimen),

5. IgG4+/IgG+ plasma cell ratio of >40%;

Most of the analyzed cases do not show all histopathologic features characteristic for IgG4-RD. The presence of two or more of the parameters listed above suggests the diagnosis of IgG4-RD [1].

The inflammatory infiltrate in IgG4-related diseases primarily consists of mature plasma cells, dispersed T lymphocytes and focally aggregated macrophages. In some cases, eosinophils are observed [1].

It must be underlined that the isolated elevated IgG4+ plasma cell count is nonspecific and insufficient for the diagnosis of IgG4-RD. Elevated IgG4+ plasma cell count is observed in many cancers and infectious diseases, which is why a range of detailed clinical and laboratory tests is crucial in differential diagnosis [85, 86]. Full clinician and pathologist cooperation is indispensable as well since incomplete patient history may delay or in some cases even prevent establishing the accurate diagnosis.

Fibrosis in IgG4-related diseases is very characteristic, being storiform with whorled or cart-wheel appearance [1, 56]. No cytologic atypia is observed within proliferating fibroblasts, which is an important element in differential diagnosis of potentially malignant lesions that may imitate IgG4-RD.

Obliterative phlebitis is the most specific but most rare histopathologic feature of IgG4-RD. In hematoxylin and eosin stained specimens a chronic intramural inflammatory infiltrate is observed with fibrosis and obliteration of the vessel lumen [1]. Elastic stain, which is a histochemical stain outlining the wall elements of the vessel damaged by the chronic inflammatory infiltration, may aid if it is difficult to accurately identify the pathologically altered and totally obliterated vein.

The accurate histopathologic diagnosis of IgG4-RD can be made when two quantity parameters for IgG4+ plasma cells are observed at the same time [4]. According to the current recommendations, the number of IgG4+ plasma cells should be determined within three high-power fields with the highest density of IgG4+ plasma cells and then the average should be determined based on three measurements [1]. For the core-needle biopsy specimen the minimal number of IgG4+ plasma cells is 10/HPF and one of the two histopathologic parameters (storiform fibrosis and/or obliterative phlebitis) must be observed. Different cutoffs are used for postoperative material, for example the cutoff within the resected salivary gland is >100 IgG4+ plasma cells/HPF [1, 56].

The key parameter, apart from elevated number of IgG4+ plasma cells is the accurate determination of IgG4+ plasma cells/total number of IgG+ plasma cells ratio. It is only the ratio of >40% that may suggest the diagnosis of IgG4-RD. The isolated elevated IgG4+ plasma cell number not accompanied by the required increase of IgG4+/IgG+ ratio does not meet the criteria for the diagnosis of IgG4-RD.

It must be stressed that plasma cells in IgG4-RD are polytypical. If a monotypical population of plasma cells is identified (even if it meets IgG4-RD criteria), a more extended histopathologic diagnosis for plasmacytic neoplasms is required—it is necessary to perform immunohistochemical staining for potential lambda and kappa light chains restriction [87].

From the point of view of histopathology and histopathologic-clinical correlations, three categories of diagnosis were enumerated [1, 56]:

- histologically highly suggestive of IgG4-RD;
- probable histologic features of IgG4-RD; and
- insufficient histopathologic evidence of IgG4-RD.

The diagnosis of "histologically highly suggestive of IgG4-RD" requires the presence of a typical storiform fibrosis or obliterative phlebitis with a high number of IgG4+ plasma cells and elevated IgG4/IgG ratio.

Histopathologic diagnosis of "probable histologic features of IgG4-RD" is based only on a high number and elevated global percentage of IgG4+ plasma cells with the lack of typical storiform fibrosis or obliterative phlebitis. A detailed correlation with clinical, laboratory and radiological data is necessary.

The third histopathologic category ("insufficient histopathologic evidence of IgG4-RD") is applied when microscopic examination does not show dense lymphoplasmacytic inflammatory infiltrate, storiform fibrosis, obliterative phlebitis or elevated number of IgG4+ plasma cells. It must be remembered though, that such diagnosis does not preclude IgG4-RD in a given patient since the primary lesion may not have been represented in the specimen taken for evaluation [1, 56].

The histopathological features of IgG4-RD in liver biopsy (**Figures** 2-5).

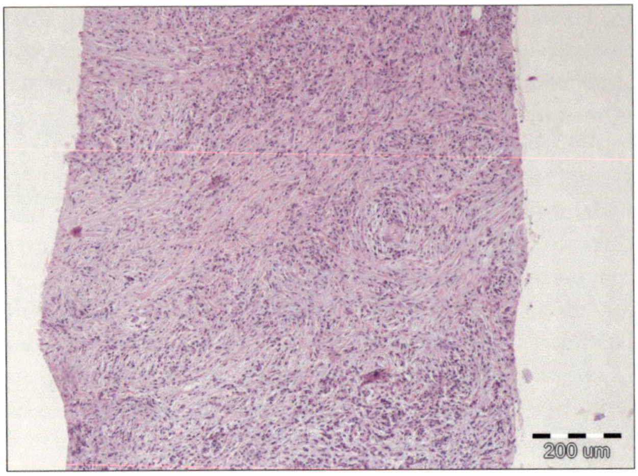

Figure 2.
Extensive fibrosis with storiform appearance and chronic inflammatory infiltrate (H&E, 200×).

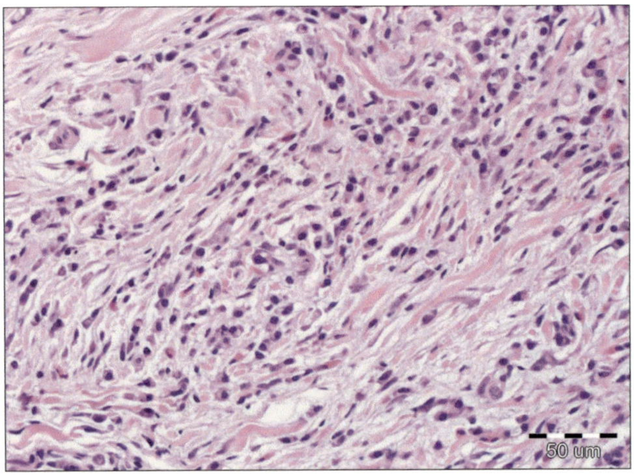

Figure 3.
Extensive fibrosis with storiform appearance and chronic inflammatory infiltrate (H&E, 400×).

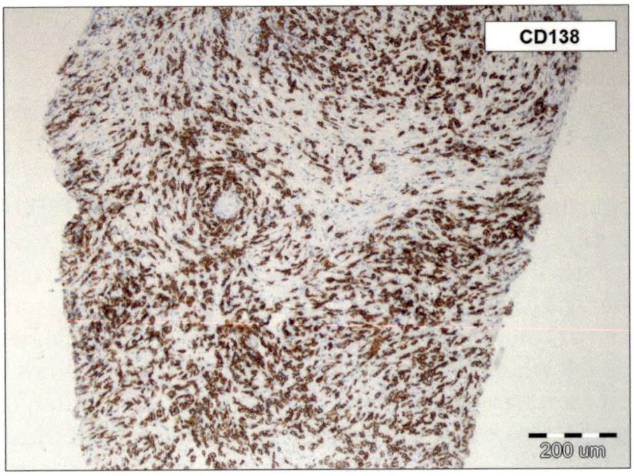

Figure 4.
Immunohistochemical staining for CD138 revealed that majority of the cells are plasmocytes (hematoxylin, 200×).

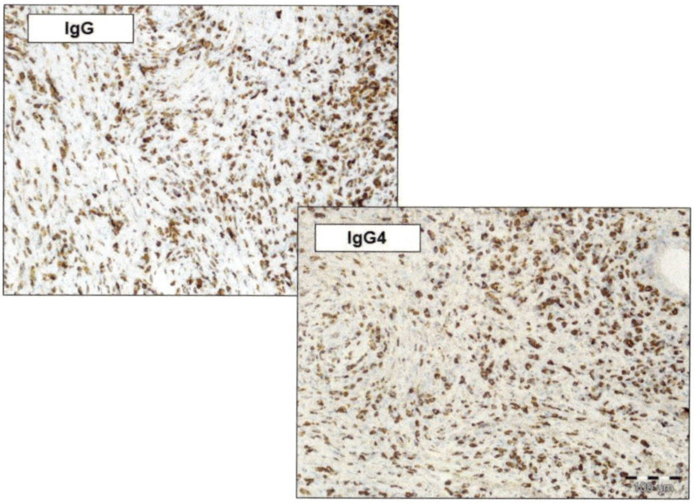

Figure 5.
A prominent component of IgG4+ plasmocytes (hematoxylin, 100×).

8. Treatment

Treatment of IgG4-RD is based on the experience of the attending physicians and opinions of the experts, as there are no large controlled clinical trials covering this problem so far. Moreover, the exact molecular pathomechanism of IgG4-RD is not known, so determination of targeted therapies is not possible at the moment. In every patient, treatment should be individually planned, depending on the location and organ damage, coexisting diseases and contraindications to immunosuppressive treatment. Another aspect of IgG4-RD therapy is that the disease tends to recur in case of treatment withdrawal. In the group of patients with the highest recurrence rate, increased baseline level of serum IgG4, IgE and eosinophils was observed [5]. At present, the experts recommend pharmacologic treatment in patients with active lymphoplasmatic infiltrations in histopathological examination. Surgery may be considered in patients with a long-lasting disease with predominant fibrosis, poorly responding to basic treatment [13, 83]. Therapy including careful observation without rapid initiation of treatment may be considered in moderate lymphadenopathy and with moderate enlargement of the submandibular salivary gland. In case of subclinical forms with involvement of the bile ducts, kidneys, aorta, retroperitoneal fibrosis, pancreas, pachymeningitis, pericarditis, treatment must be started even with a lack of clinical symptoms due to progressive, irreversible organ damage.

According to international guidelines of IgG4-RD treatment, the first-line medicines are glucocorticoids: oral prednisone, at an initial dose of 0.6 mg/kg daily maintained for 2–4 weeks and gradually reduced for 3–6 months [83, 84]. In Japanese guidelines, glucocorticoids in small maintenance doses (5–10 mg daily) are recommended even for 3 years [88]. In case of recurrences, repeated administration of glucocorticoids is proposed in the above schedule [83]. Most of the patients show fast improvement after glucocorticoid use. As soon as after several weeks of treatment, improvement of functional parameters of the involved organs is observed, with a reduction of the infiltration mass and a decrease of serum IgG4 concentration.

There are no publications which would constitute guidelines for the application of disease modifying antirheumatic drugs in patients not responding to or not tolerating treatment with glucocorticoids or who experience frequent disease recurrences. In 46% of patients with IgG4-RD who have their glucocorticoid doses decreased, the disease recurs [89]. As in other rheumatic diseases, the disease modifying antirheumatic drugs are tried in such cases. The adjunctive therapy has so far applied most drugs used in rheumatology, including methotrexate, azathioprine, mycophenolate mofetil, cyclophosphamide. However, the results and their efficacy are different. Adjunctive treatment with disease modifying antirheumatic drugs is currently based mainly on the experience of attending physicians and is experimental. At present, there are no well-designed clinical trials summarizing this problem. Moreover, the disease modifying antirheumatic drugs were always used as adjunctive treatment to glucocorticoid therapy and not as first-line therapy, therefore their efficacy is even more difficult to evaluate. In 2017, a summary of observations in patients treated with glucocorticoids vs. glucocorticoids and cyclophosphamide orally was published [90]. It turned out that a combination of disease modifying antirheumatic drugs decreased the risk of disease recurrence by 70% as compared to the group treated with glucocorticoid monotherapy.

In case vascular location and lesions in the aorta, there are no explicit guidelines concerning treatment. Similarly as in other forms of IgG4-RD, steroids are used, most commonly prednisone at a dose of 0.6 mg/kg daily. This dose is gradually reduced to the maintenance dose of 5 mg/kg daily. There are no guidelines concerning therapy duration. Steroid administration does not protect against development and progression of aneurysms in patients in whom vascular wall widening was found initially [9, 80]. In this group of patients, surgery is performed in case of confirmation of indications by vascular surgeons.

Due to participation of T and B lymphocytes in the pathomechanism of the disease, the first biological drug which turned out to be effective in the treatment of IgG4-RD was rituximab (RTX). Typically this drug is used intravenously at a dose of 1 g every 15 days, up to a dose of 2 g [91]. In a prospective open-label clinical trial, RTX was effective in 97% of patients with IgG4-RD after 6 months of therapy despite no glucocorticoids used [80]. Also, the efficacy of RTX in patients with involvement of cerebrospinal meninges was reported on [92]. Currently RTX is recommended by experts for use as a second-line therapy in patients with recurrent disease or not responding to basic treatment [92].

So far, the data from a clinical trial with XmAB5871, i.e., a reversible inhibitor of CD19+ on B lymphocytes, were not published.

The patients with IgG4-RD are shown in **Figure 6**, before and after treatment.

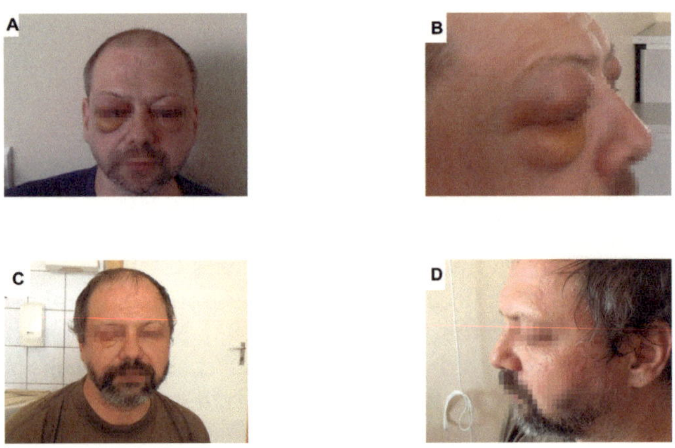

Figure 6.
Typical Mikulicz disease (IgG4-related disease) with lacrimal enlargement at the diagnosis (A, B) and after 10 months of treatment (C, D) with prednison 0.6 mg/kg/day.

9. Evaluation of disease activity and efficacy of the therapy

For evaluation of disease activity and efficacy of the therapy, IgG4 Responder index is used. This index includes 25 domains, regarding organ location of lesions and general symptoms. For every domain, 0 to 3 scores may be assigned. The disease is active if the index score is 3 or higher [93].

The prognosis regarding IgG4-RD is not known. There are no long-term, well-designed observational studies. It seems that spontaneous remissions rarely occur. However, the disease recurrences are frequently observed when glucocorticoids are reduced. The disease, if not diagnosed, may lead to irreversible fibrosis and damage of the involved organs. It should be remembered that due to the diversity of clinical pictures in IgG4-RD, all physicians may encounter this entity in their practice, regardless of their specialty.

Conflict of interest

None declare.

Author details

Agata Sebastian[1]*, Piotr Donizy[2] and Piotr Wiland[1]

1 Department of Rheumatology and Internal Medicine,
Wroclaw Medical University, Wroclaw, Poland

2 Department of Pathomorphology and Oncological Cytology,
Wroclaw Medical University, Wroclaw, Poland

*Address all correspondence to: agatasebastian@vp.pl

References

[1] Bledsoe JR, Della-Torre E, Rovati L, et al. IgG4-related disease: review of the histopathologic features, differential diagnosis, and therapeutic approach. APMIS. 2018;**126**(6):459-476

[2] Bozzalla Cassione E, Stone JH. IgG4-related disease. Current Opinion in Rheumatology. 2017;**29**(3):223-227

[3] Kamisawa T, Egawa N, Nakajima H. Autoimmune pancreatitis is a systemic autoimmune disease. The American Journal of Gastroenterology. 2003;**98**:2811-2812

[4] Stone JH, Khosroshahi A, Deshpande V, et al. Recommendations for the nomenclature of IgG4-related disease and its individual organ system manifestations. Arthritis and Rheumatism. 2012;**64**(10):3061-3067

[5] Stone JH. IgG4-related disease: Nomenclature, clinical features, and treatment. Seminars in Diagnostic Pathology. 2012;**29**(4):177-190

[6] Uchida K, Masamune A, Shimosegawa T, et al. Prevalence of IgG4-related disease in Japan based on nationwide survey in 2009. International Journal of Rheumatology. 2012;**2012**:358-371

[7] Umehara H, Okazaki K, Nakamura T, et al. Current approach to the diagnosis of IgG4-related disease—Combination of comprehensivediagnostic and organ-specific criteria. Modern Rheumatology. 2017;**27**(3):381-391

[8] Karim F, Loeffen J, Bramer W, et al. IgG4-related disease: A systematic review of this unrecognized disease in pediatrics. Pediatric Rheumatology Online Journal. 2016;**14**(1):18

[9] Kasashima F, Kawakami K, Matsumoto Y, et al. IgG4-related arterial disease. Annals of Vascular Diseases. 2018;**11**(1):72-77

[10] Inoue D, Yoshida K, Yoneda N, et al. IgG4-related disease: Dataset of 235 consecutive patients. Medicine. 2015;**94**:e680

[11] Perugino CA, Wallace ZS, Meyersohn N, et al. Large vessel involvement by IgG4-related disease. Medicine. 2016;**95**:e3344

[12] Della-Torre E, Lanzillotta M, Doglioni C. Immunology of IgG4-related disease. Clinical and Experimental Immunology. 2015;**181**(2):191-206

[13] Della-Torre E, Feeney E, Deshpande V, et al. B-cell depletion attenuates serological biomarkers of fibrosis and myofibroblast activation in IgG4-related disease. Annals of the Rheumatic Diseases. 2015;**74**(12):2236-2243

[14] Saito Y, Kagami S, Kawashima S, et al. Roles of CRTH2+ CD4+ T cells in immunoglobulin G4-related lacrimal gland enlargement. International Archives of Allergy and Immunology. 2012;**158**(Suppl 1):42-46

[15] Zen Y, Fujii T, Harada K, Kawano M, et al. Th2 and regulatory immune reactions are increased in immunoglobin G4-related sclerosing pancreatitis and cholangitis. Hepatology. 2007;**45**(6):1538-1546

[16] Mattoo H, Della-Torre E, Mahajan VS, et al. Circulating Th2 memory cells in IgG4-related disease are restricted to a defined subset of subjects with atopy. Allergy. 2014;**69**(3):399-402

[17] Carruthers MN, Khosroshahi A, Augustin T, et al. The diagnostic utility of serum IgG4 concentrations in IgG4-related disease. Annals of the Rheumatic Diseases. 2015;**74**(1):14-18

[18] Chen Y, Zhao JZ, Feng RE, et al. Types of organ involvement in patients with immunoglobulin G4-related disease. Chinese Medical Journal. 2016;**129**:1525-1532

[19] You C, Della Torre E, Mattoo H, et al. Prevalence of atopy, eosinophilia, and IgE elevation in IgG4-related disease. Allergy. 2014;**69**:269-272

[20] Akiyama M, Yasuoka H, Yamaoka K, et al. Enhanced IgG4 production by follicular helper 2 T cells and the involvement of follicular helper 1 T cells in the pathogenesis of IgG4-related disease. Arthritis Research & Therapy. 2016;**13**(18):167

[21] Akiyama M, Suzuki K, Yamaoka K, et al. Number of circulating follicular helper 2 T cells correlates with IgG4 and interleukin-4 levels and plasmablast numbers in IgG4-related disease. Arthritis & Rhematology. 2015;**67**(9):2476-2481

[22] Vasaitis L. IgG4-related disease: A relatively new concept for clinicians. European Journal of Internal Medicine. 2016;**27**:1-9

[23] Wallace ZS, Mattoo H, Carruthers M, et al. Plasmablasts as a biomarker for IgG4-related disease, independent of serum IgG4concentrations. Annals of the Rheumatic Diseases. 2015;**74**(1):190-195

[24] Morita R, Schmitt N, Bentebibel SE, et al. Human blood CXCR5(+)CD4(+) T cells are counterparts of T follicular cells and contain specific subsets that differentially support antibody secretion. Immunity. 2011;**34**:108-121

[25] Grados A, Ebbo M, Piperoglou C, et al. T cell polarization toward Th2/Tfh2 and Th17/Tfh17 in patients with IgG4-related disease. Frontiers in Immunology. 2017;**8**:235

[26] Miyoshi H, Uchida K, Taniguchi T, et al. Circulating na€ıve and CD4+ CD25high regulatory T cells in patients with autoimmune pancreatitis. Pancreas. 2008;**36**:133-140

[27] Mattoo H, Della-Torre E, Mahajan VS, et al. Circulating Th2 memory cells in IgG4-related disease are restricted to a defined subset ofsubjects with atopy. Allergy. 2014;**69**:399-402

[28] Mattoo H, Stone JH, Pillai S. Clonally expanded cytotoxic CD4+ T cells and the pathogenesis of IgG4-related disease. Autoimmunity. 2017;**50**:19-24

[29] Mattoo H, Mahajan VS, Maehara T, et al. Clonal expansion of CD4(+) cytotoxic T lymphocytes in patients with IgG4-related disease. The Journal of Allergy and Clinical Immunology. 2016;**138**:825-838

[30] Hubers LM, Vos H, Schuurman AR, et al. Annexin A11 is targeted by IgG4 and IgG1 autoantibodies in IgG4-related disease. Gut. 2018;**67**:728-735

[31] Nirula A, Glaser SM, Kalled SL, et al. What is IgG4? A review of the biology of a unique immunoglobulin subtype. Current Opinion in Rheumatology. 2011;**23**:119-124

[32] Lichtenstein LM, Holtzman NA, Burnett LS. A quantitative in vitro study of the chromatographic distribution and immunoglobulin characteristics of human blocking antibody. Journal of Immunology. 1968;**101**(2):317-324

[33] James LK, Bowen H, Calvert RA, Dodev TS, Shamji MH, Beavil AJ, et al. Allergen specificity of IgG(4)-expressing B cells in patients with grass pollen allergy undergoing immunotherapy. The Journal of Allergy and Clinical Immunology. 2012;**130**(3):663-670

[34] Koneczny IA. New classification system for IgG4 autoantibodies. Frontiers in Immunology. 2018;**12**(9):97

[35] Aalberse RC, Stapel SO, Schuurman J, Rispens T. Immunoglobulin G4: An odd antibody. Clinical and Experimental Allergy. 2009;**39**:469-477

[36] Umehara H, Okazaki K, Masaki Y, et al. A novel clinical entity, IgG4-related disease (IgG4RD): General concept and details. Modern Rheumatology. 2012;**22**:1-14

[37] Legatowicz-Koprowska M. IgG4-related disease: Why is it so important? Central European Journal of Immunology. 2018;**43**(2):204-208

[38] Wallace ZS, Khosroshahi A, Carruthers MD, et al. An international multispecialty validation study of the IgG4-related disease responder index. Arthritis Care & Research. 2018;**70**(11):1671-1678

[39] Sarkar A, Pitchumoni CS. The protean manifestations of IgG4-RD in gastrointestinal disorders. Disease-a-Month. 2015;**61**(12):493-515

[40] Zhang Z, Fu W, Wang M, et al. IgG4-related inflammatory pseudotumor of the brain parenchyma: A case report and literature review. Acta Neurologica Belgica. 2018;**118**(4):617-627

[41] Sebastian A, Sebastian M, Misterska-Skóra M, et al. The variety of clinical presentations in IgG4-related disease in rheumatology. Rheumatology International. 2018;**38**(2):303-309

[42] Mart_ınez-Valle F, Fern_andez-Codina A, Pinal-Fern_andez I, et al. IgG4-related disease: Evidence from six recent cohorts. Autoimmunity Reviews. 2017;**16**:168-172

[43] Yamamoto M, Takahashi H, Shinomura Y. Mechanisms and assessment of IgG4-related disease: Lessons for the rheumatologist. Nature Reviews Rheumatology. 2014;**10**:148-159

[44] Umehara H, Okazaki K, Masaki Y, et al. Comprehensive diagnostic criteria for IgG4-related disease (IgG4-RD), 2011. Modern Rheumatology. 2012;**22**(1):21-30

[45] Yamamoto M, Tabeya T, Naishiro Y, et al. Value of serum IgG4 in the diagnosis of IgG4-related disease and in differentiation from rheumatic diseases and other diseases. Modern Rheumatology. 2012;**22**(3):419-425

[46] Mavragani CP, Fragoulis GE, Rontogianni D, et al. Elevated IgG4 serum levels among primary Sjögren's syndrome patients: Do they unmask underlying IgG4-related disease? Arthritis Care and Research. 2014;**66**:773-777

[47] Chen LF, Mo YQ, Ma JD, et al. Elevated serum IgG4 defines specific clinical phenotype of rheumatoid arthritis. Mediators of Inflammation. 2014;**2014**:635293. DOI: 10.1155/2014/635293

[48] Yamamoto M, Yajima H, Takahashi H, et al. Everyday clinical practice in IgG4-related dacryoadenitis and/or sialadenitis: Results from the SMART database. Modern Rheumatology. 2015;**25**:199-204

[49] Cheuk W, Yuen HK, Chan AC, et al. Ocular adnexal lymphoma associated with IgG4 + chronic sclerosing dacryoadenitis: A previously undescribed complication of IgG4-related sclerosing disease. The American Journal of Surgical Pathology. 2008;**32**:1159-1167

[50] Venkataraman G, Rizzo KA, Chavez JJ, et al. Marginal zone lymphomas involving meningeal dura: Possible link to IgG4-related diseases. Modern Pathology. 2011;**24**:355-366

[51] Hart PA, Law RJ, Dierkhising R, et al. Risk of cancer in autoimmune

pancreatitis: A case-control study and review of the literature. Pancreas. 2014;**43**:417-421

[52] Hirano K, Tada M, Sasahira N, et al. Incidence of malignancies in patients with IgG4-related disease. Internal Medicine. 2014;**53**:171-176

[53] Zheng K, Teng F, Li XM. Immunoglobulin G4-related kidney disease: Pathogenesis, diagnosis, and treatment. Chronic Diseases and Translational Medicine. 2017;**3**(3):138-114

[54] Abraham M, Khosroshahi A. Diagnostic and treatment workup for IgG4-related disease. Expert Review of Clinical Immunology. 2017;**13**(9):867-875

[55] Mahajan VS, Mattoo H, Deshpande V, et al. IgG4-related disease. Annual Review of Pathology. 2014;**9**:315-347

[56] Deshpande V, Zen Y, Chan JK, et al. Consensus statement on the pathology of IgG4-related disease. Modern Pathology. 2012;**25**:1181-1192

[57] Deshpande V. IgG4 related disease of the head and neck. Head and Neck Pathology. 2015;**9**(1):24-31

[58] Sah RP, Chari ST. Clinical hypothyroidism in autoimmune pancreatitis. Pancreas. 2010;**39**:1114-1116

[59] Kottahachchi D, Topliss DJ. Immunoglobulin G4-related thyroid diseases. European Thyroid Journal. 2016;**5**(4):231-239

[60] Li Y, Nishihara E, Hirokawa M, et al. Distinct clinical, serological, and sonographic characteristics of Hashimoto's thyroiditis based with and without IgG4-positive plasma cells. The Journal of Clinical Endocrinology and Metabolism. 2010;**95**(3):1309-1317

[61] Kasashima S, Kawashima A, Kasashima F, et al. Inflammatory features, including symptoms, increased serum interleukin-6, and C-reactive protein, in IgG4-related vascular diseases. Heart and Vessels. 2018. DOI: 10.1007/s00380-018-1203-8

[62] Matsui S, Yamamoto H, Minamoto S, et al. Proposed diagnostic criteria for IgG4-related respiratory disease. Respiratory Investigation. 2016;**54**(2):130-132

[63] Brito-Zerón P, Ramos-Casals M, Bosch X, et al. The clinical spectrum of IgG4-related disease. Autoimmunity Reviews. 2014;**13**(12):1203-1210

[64] Ghazale A, Chari ST, Zhang L, et al. Immunoglobulin G4-associated cholangitis: Clinical profile and response to therapy. Gastroenterology. 2008;**134**(3):706-715

[65] Kamisawa T, Nakajima H, Egawa N, et al. IgG4-related sclerosing disease incorporating sclerosing pancreatitis, cholangitis, sialadenitis and retroperitoneal fibrosis with lymphadenopathy. Pancreatology. 2006;**6**(1-2):132-137

[66] Matsubayashi H, Sawai H, Kimura H, et al. Characteristics of autoimmune pancreatitis based on serum IgG4 level. Digestive and Liver Disease. 2011;**43**(9):731-735

[67] Patel H, Khalili K, Kyoung KT, et al. IgG4 related disease—Aretrospective descriptive study highlighting Canadian experiences in diagnosis and management. BMC Gastroenterology. 2013;**13**:168

[68] Okazaki K, Uchida K. Current concept of autoimmune pancreatitis and IgG4-related disease. The American Journal of Gastroenterology. 2018;**113**(10):1412-1416

[69] Raissian Y, Nasr SH, Larsen CP, et al. Diagnosis of IgG4-related tubulointerstitial nephritis. Journal of the American Society of Nephrology. 2011;**22**(7):1343-1352

[70] Salvadori M, Tsalouchos A. Immunoglobulin G4-related kidney diseases: An updated review. World Journal of Nephrology. 2018;**7**(1):29-40

[71] Zhang P, Cornell LD. IgG4-related tubulointerstitial nephritis. Advances in Chronic Kidney Disease. 2017;**24**:94-100

[72] Stone JH, Brito-Zerón P, Bosch X, Ramos-Casals M. Diagnostic approach to the complexity of IgG4-related disease. Mayo Clinic Proceedings. 2015;**90**:927-939

[73] Saeki T, Nishi S, Imai N, Ito T, Yamazaki H, Kawano M, et al. Clinicopathological characteristics of patients with IgG4-related tubulointerstitial nephritis. Kidney International. 2010;**78**:1016-1023

[74] Saeki T, Kawano M. IgG4-related kidney disease. Kidney International. 2014;**85**(2):251-257

[75] Walker DI, Bloor K, Williams G, et al. Inflammatory aneurysms of the abdominal aorta. The British Journal of Surgery. 1972;**59**:609-614

[76] Kasashima S, Zen Y, Kawashima A, et al. A clinicopathologic study of immunoglobulin G4-related sclerosing disease of the thoracic aorta. Journal of Vascular Surgery. 2010;**52**:1587-1595

[77] Stone JH, Khosroshahi A, Deshpande V, et al. IgG4-related systemic disease accounts for a significant proportion of thoracic lymphoplasmacytic aortitis cases. Arthritis Care & Research. 2010;**62**:316-322

[78] Ebbo M, Daniel L, Pavic M, et al. IgG4-related systemic disease: Features and treatment response in a French cohort: Results of a multicenterregistry. Medicine (Baltimore). 2012;**91**(1):49-56

[79] Toyoda K, Oba H, Kutomi K, et al. MR imaging of IgG4-related disease in the head and neck and brain. AJNR. American Journal of Neuroradiology. 2012;**33**(11):2136-2139

[80] Carruthers MN, Topazian MD, Khosroshahi A, et al. Rituximab for IgG4-related disease: A prospective, open-label trial. Annals of the Rheumatic Diseases. 2015;**74**(6):1171-1177

[81] Takayama R, Ueno T, Saeki H. Immunoglobulin G4-related disease and its skin manifestations. The Journal of Dermatology. 2017;**44**(3):288-296

[82] Tokura Y, Yagi H, Yanaguchi H, et al. IgG4-related skin disease. The British Journal of Dermatology. 2014;**171**(5):959-967

[83] Khosroshahi A, Carruthers MN, Stone JH, et al. Rethinking Ormond's disease: "Idiopathic" retroperitoneal fibrosis in the era of IgG4-related disease. Medicine (Baltimore). 2013;**92**(2):82-91

[84] Stone JH. Aortitis, retroperitoneal fibrosis, and IgG4-related disease. Presse Médicale. 2013;**42**(4 Pt 2): 622-625

[85] Deshpande V. The pathology of IgG4-related disease: Critical issues and challenges. Seminars in Diagnostic Pathology. 2012;**29**:191-196

[86] Strehl JD, Hartmann A, Agaimy A. Numerous IgG4-positive plasma cells are ubiquitous in diverse localised non-specific chronic inflammatory conditions and need to be distinguished from IgG4-related systemic disorders. Journal of Clinical Pathology. 2011;**64**:237-243

[87] Ferry JA. IgG4-related lymphadenopathy and IgG4-related lymphoma: Moving targets. Diagnostic Histopathology. 2013;**19**:128-139

[88] Khosroshahi A, Wallace ZS, Crowe JL, et al. International consensus guidance statement on the management and treatment of IgG4-related disease. Arthritis & Rhematology. 2015;**67**:1688-1699

[89] Okazaki K, Kawa S, Kamisawa T, et al. Amendment of the Japanese Consensus Guidelines for Autoimmune Pancreatitis, 2013. I. Concept and diagnosis of autoimmune pancreatitis. Journal of Gastroenterology. 2014;**49**:567-588

[90] Yunyun F, Yu C, Panpan Z, et al. Efficacy of cyclophosphamide treatment for immunoglobulin G4-related disease with addition of glucocorticoids. Scientific Reports. 2017;**21**:6195

[91] Ebbo M, Grados A, Samson M, et al. Long-term efficacy and safety of rituximab in IgG4-related disease: Data from a French nationwide study of thirty-three patients. PLoS One. 2017;**12**(9):e0183844

[92] Akiyama M, Takeuchi T. IgG4-related disease: Beyond glucocorticoids. Drugs & Aging. 2018;**35**(4):275-287

[93] Carruthers MN, Stone JH, Deshpande V, et al. Development of an IgG4-RD responder index. International Journal of Rheumatology. 2012;**2012**:259408

Chapter 6

Autoimmune Pancreatitis: Clinical Presentation and Therapy

Zoltán Berger Fleiszig and Carla Mancilla Asencio

Abstract

Autoimmune pancreatitis is a relatively recently identified entity. The dominant type 1 is the pancreatic manifestation of a systemic IgG4-related fibroinflammatory disease. The type 2 has a clearly different histology, its dominant feature is a granulocytic epithelial lesion, and it is independent of IgG4. While type 1 is rather a disease with male dominance in majors than 50-year-old people, no gender difference is observed in type 2, and the disease is more frequently seen in young people. The more frequent initial clinical manifestation is obstructive jaundice in type 1, while abdominal pain and mild acute pancreatitis in type 2. CT and magnetic resonance images are very similar, IgG4 can be normal even in type 1, and the associated involvement of other organs is frequently posterior to the pancreatic manifestation; thus, the distinction of the two types of AIP can be difficult without histology in the everyday clinical practice. Several cases can be undetermined and qualified as Not Otherwise Specified (NOS). However, all types of AIP respond quickly to steroid treatment with a complete recovery. Late prognosis is good, but up to 50% recurrence has been observed in type 1, and several authors have described progression to chronic pancreatitis.

Keywords: autoimmune pancreatitis, IgG4-related disease, granulocytic epithelial lesion, histology, steroid treatment, complete recovery

1. Introduction

Autoimmune pancreatitis (AIP) is an emerging disease, recognized with an increasing frequency in the whole world. Autoimmune factors have been known since long time to participate in the etiology of some cases of chronic pancreatitis [1]; however, their importance was somewhat marginal, no more than 3–5% of the patients of chronic pancreatitis [2, 3]. In addition, pancreatic involvement is relatively rare in the major autoimmune diseases: while described, chronic pancreatitis is only exceptionally found in lupus erythematosus [4] and Sjögren's syndrome [5, 6]. Conversely, AIP while described before [7, 8] was identified as an independent entity only in 1995 [9], and it is associated with specific IgG4-related autoimmune disease (type 1) and with inflammatory bowel disease (type 2). Their histology is characteristic and quite different when compared to pancreatic involvement in SLE or Sjögren's syndrome. This fact is very similar to the case of the liver, hepatitis associated with lupus and autoimmune hepatitis being also the two distinct diseases [10].

2. Definition, classification, and histology

The concept of autoimmune pancreatitis was introduced by Yoshida in 1995 [9] and accepted worldwide. The majority of cases initially described came from Asia, but later on the disease was recognized in the whole world. With the exponentially growing information, two different forms were distinguished: the type 1 or lymphoplasmacytic sclerosing pancreatitis (LPSP) and the type 2 or idiopathic duct-centric pancreatitis. Type 1 has been dominant in the whole world and represents the most frequent digestive manifestation of a systemic fibroinflammatory IgG4-related disease. Its histology is characteristic: the association of storiform fibrosis, obliterative phlebitis, and marked lymphoplasmacytic infiltration are unique, and the immunohistology can be the final proof, demonstrating the presence of more than 40% of IgG4-positive lymphocytes as compared to the whole number of IgG-positive cells. Details of the autoimmune reaction are well described, but the whole process is not known. Circulating plasmablasts are present in increased number in the active phase of the disease and decrease rapidly with the treatment [11]. Interaction of T- and B lymphocytes has been demonstrated. Th2 reaction and regulator T-cell activation are part of the process, resulting from one part in an increase of interleukins 4, 5, and 13 with a consecutive increase of eosinophils and serum IgE and from the other part increased IL-10 production, lymphoplasmacytes, and fibroblast proliferation, with an increased IgG4 level. As these diseases are recognized as IgG4-related, one could expect IgG4 lymphoplasmacytes as key factors inducing the immune reaction and organ damage. However, the characteristics of the IgG4 subclass do not permit complement activation or immune complex formation. Both IgG4 and IgG1 obtained from an active AIP patient, when injected separately, induced pancreatic damage in experimental design. However, when injected simultaneously, IgG4 was rather protective and reduced the IgG1-induced pancreatic damage [12]. Based on these experimental data, IgG1 subclass seems to be more active in producing damage, and the local increase of IgG4 cells and elevated serum IgG4 level seems to be rather a consequence. In type 2, AIP has a clearly different histology. The fibrosis is important, but not storiform, phlebitis/venulitis is rare, and if present, it is not obliterative. The essential finding is infiltration by neutrophil leucocytes, forming the typical granulocytic epithelial lesion (GEL), with duct cell damage. Similar lesions can also be observed in pancreatic lobules. While lymphoplasmacytic infiltration can exist, IgG4-positive cells are rare. A unique finding in type 2. AIP is the presence of IL-8 around the ductal cells, in particular in the damaged pancreatic ducts. IL-8 is a chemotactic factor for neutrophils, and its high expression is in line with the formation of granulocytic epithelial lesions [13]. In addition, similar accumulation of IL-8 was described in the damaged mucosa of ulcerative colitis but not in other types of colitis. This finding points out a similarity in pathomechanism of these diseases as a possible explanation of the well-known association.

2.1 Autoantibodies: serology

Several autoantibodies were described in AIP, against carbonic anhydrase [14] and amylase [15], but they do not have any demonstrated role in the initiation of the autoimmune process. A cross-reaction was found against a protein of *Helicobacter*, the plasminogen-binding protein [16], but its role in the pathogenesis of AIP was not confirmed. Unspecific autoantibodies, as antinuclear and anti-DNA, can also be present. A variety of autoantibodies have been found in the sera of patients with AIP, but none of these autoantibodies appear to be disease specific. The serum IgG4 level has been found elevated in a variable proportion of confirmed type 1 AIP cases. Sensitivity above 80% was published in some papers, while others found only

<50% [17]. On the contrary, IgG4 can be elevated even in some cases of pancreatic cancer. Once increased, the serum IgG4 level is a useful marker in confirming the diagnosis of AIP type 1, but a normal value does not exclude AIP. Unfortunately, no specific test exists even for the diagnosis of AIP type 1, and type 2 is not accompanied by laboratory alterations. In our experience [18], we found IgG4 > 135 mg% in 80% of confirmed AIP type 1 cases but in none of 20 NOS undetermined cases, while several of these patients, if not the majority of them, were probably seronegative type 1. It means that the real diagnostic performance was far less than 80% in our clinical practice, even considering a lower cutoff value.

3. Epidemiology and clinical characteristics

AIP is increasingly recognized. For example, 900 cases were known in Japan in 2002 [19]; 2790 in 2007 [20]; and 5745 in 2011 [21]. The calculated prevalence was 4.6/100,000, while the incidence 1.4/100,000/yr. Experiences from different regions of the world have been increasingly published; the annual number of papers increased exponentially from 39 in 2000 to 935 in 2017, as found in PubMed Central. We also observed a marked increase in the diagnosis of AIP in Chile [18]. However, the worldwide increase in the frequency of this disease is probably mainly due to its better recognition rather than a-so-important increase in incidence. The more frequent type 1 AIP is part of a systemic IgG4- related disease. A male dominance has been observed; about two thirds of patients are men. The average age is above 50 years. However, there are also women in considerable number. The pancreatic affection is frequently associated with manifestation of the same disease in other organs. Recurrence in the pancreas or in other organs is relatively frequent in this form. Type 2 AIP has been described later, but it is also recognized with a growing frequency. No gender difference was described, and the disease affects young people; the mean age is no more than 30 years. The only associated disease is inflammatory bowel disease (IBD), mainly ulcerative colitis, which can occur simultaneously with the pancreatitis or any other period, before or after the AIP. This form of pancreatitis seldom recurs (**Table 1**)

	Type 1 (LPSP)	**Type 2 (IDCP)**
Sex	Male dominance (two to three times)	No difference
Age	After fifth decade	Young people, <30
Dominant symptom	Jaundice	Pain, mild pancreatitis
Serum IgG4 level	Frequently increased (50–80%)	Normal
Associated diseases	IgG4-related organ involvement	Inflammatory bowel disease
Response to steroids	Quick, complete	Quick, complete
Relapse	>30%	Rare, <10%

LPSP, lymphoplasmacytic sclerosing pancreatitis; IDCP, idiopathic duct-centric pancreatitis.

Table 1.
Clinical characteristics of two types of autoimmune pancreatitis.

4. Diagnosis

4.1 Clinical symptoms

The clinical manifestation of AIP is variable and non-specific. The most frequent symptom is painless jaundice due to compression of intrapancreatic segment of choledochus by the fibroinflammatory process in the pancreatic head. Unfortunately, it shares typical symptoms of pancreatic head cancer and represents one of the most challenging difficulties in differential diagnosis. Abdominal pain and mild acute pancreatitis are also important manifestations. However, severe acute pancreatitis and major local fluid collections practically do not occur and autoimmunity is not a frequent cause of recurrent acute pancreatitis.

4.2 Serology

As described above, the only valuable serological marker is the serum IgG4 level [17]. However, its performance in the diagnosis is variable: it can be increased only in type 1, not in type 2. Other unspecific autoantibodies have low sensibility in AIP and are not used routinely. Sometimes, IgE and peripheral eosinophils can be increased. If altered, they help in the diagnosis; if not, they have no value in excluding it.

4.3 Images

Radiologic exams, CT scan, and MR are the bases of the diagnosis in the everyday clinical practice [22]. Typical sausage-like increase in pancreatic size with a peripheral halo is seen in several cases when the pancreas is diffusely affected. Frequently, only segments of pancreas are involved. In these cases the differences in density or signal intensity as compared to the normal segments (**Figures 1b, 2b** and **3a,b**), the late enhancement with contrast, and the irregular stricture of the main pancreatic duct can be helpful. In the difficult situation when there is a clinical suspicion of pancreatic cancer, even without a clear-cut mass, the absence of significant upstream duct dilation is an important element which

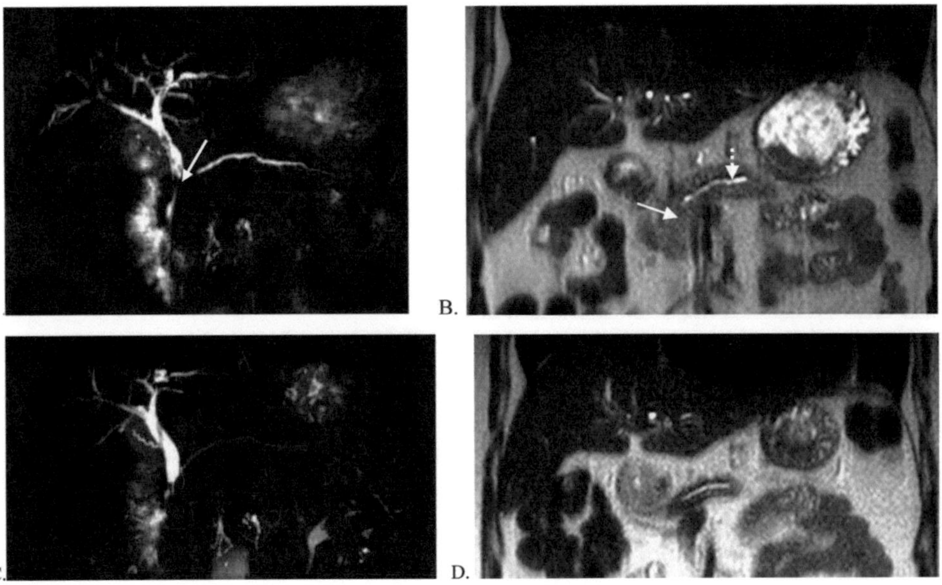

A. B. C. D.

Figure 1.
(a) Magnetic resonance cholangiography showing pancreatic duct stricture in the head and stenosis of intrapancreatic segment of choledochus with proximal dilatation. Pancreatic duct is only slightly dilated in the body and tail. (b) Pancreatic head is enlarged with slightly hyperintense signal in T2. The pancreatic duct is only seen in the body and tail. (c and d) The same patient and same images after 2 months of treatment. Almost complete recovery, with slight pancreatic atrophy. The images of this chapter come from the Radiolology Department of Clinical Hospital of University of Chile and are the authors' property.

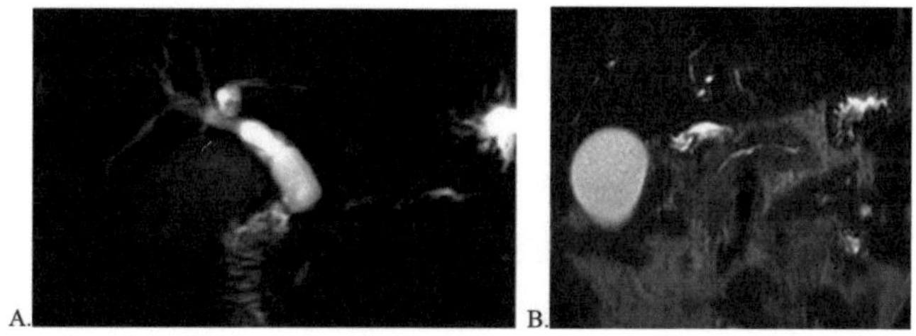

Figure 2.
(a) Markedly dilated choledochus, proximal to the stenotic intrapancreatic segment of the bile duct. Irregular multiple stenosis of the main pancreatic duct. (b) Again, the structured pancreatic duct is practically not seen in the augmented pancreatic head, but the upstream dilatation is only mild.

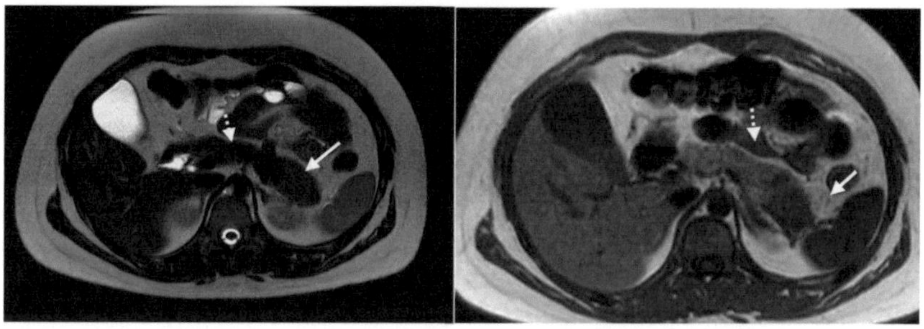

Figure 3.
Focal AIP in the pancreatic tail. (a) T2, hyperintensity of the signal; (b) T1, hypointense signal. Arrow: the swollen pancreatic segment. Pointed arrow: normal pancreas. Note the clear limitation between the normal and involved segments.

helps to distinguish the two pathologies with diametrically different prognoses (**Figures 1a,b, 2a,b** and **5a**). It is noteworthy that neither necrosis nor major peri-pancreatic fluid collection are seen in AIP. Sometimes, pseudocysts can complicate the disease [23]; they also respond to steroids and can disappear even completely. It is important to emphasize that there is no difference in the radiologic alterations in types 1 and 2 of AIP.

4.3.1 When to perform diagnostic ERCP and biliary drainage?

The necessity of ERCP in order to establish the diagnosis of AIP nowadays is an exception. Magnetic resonance images have a similar sensibility in the diagnosis. If performed, irregular and usually multifocal narrowing of the main pancreatic duct is seen in the affected pancreatic segment, without an important upstream dilatation (**Figure 5a**). Stenosis of intrapancreatic segment of choledochus is frequent, and, sometimes, irregular strictures of extra- and intrahepatic bile ducts can show the associated IgG4-related cholangitis, very similar to the primary sclerosing cholangitis (PSC) (**Figures 5b** and **6a**). The clinical need of ERCP is determined in the majority of the cases by the severe obstructive jaundice and the intention to drain the obstructed dilated bile duct with a biliary endoprosthesis (**Figures 5b** and **6b**). However, it is at least a matter of discussion: the decrease in bilirubin level in response to steroid treatment is strikingly rapid, and it seems better to avoid unnecessary instrumentalization of biliary tract with the risk of bacterial contamination. Once ERCP is performed without the previous suspicion of AIP and contrast material injected in the obstructed bile duct, stent placement is mandatory as in any other causes of bile duct obstruction. In our practice, we performed ERCP only in our first patients, later on only in some exceptional cases when even concomitant sclerosing cholangitis was not excluded, and it was impossible to avoid biliary stent placement. In fact, Chari's group published the same tendency from Mayo Clinic [24].

4.4 Other organ involvement

A type 1 AIP is a systemic disease; we can see frequently signs of the disease in other organs. Fibroinflammatory tumor-like pathology of lacrimal and salivary glands is clearly visible, palpable, and easy to access for a biopsy. However, other manifestations, as frequent bilateral nephritis, can be asymptomatic but easily detectable on the MR image (**Figure 4a**), frequently synchronic with the pancreatic disease. Peritoneal fibrosis and aortitis can occur in different times, before or later, as compared to AIP. In our experience PSC like cholangitis and bilateral multifocal nephritis were the most frequent extrapancreatic manifestations, found in 8 and 11 of our 44 type 1 patients, respectively [18]. Any of these manifestations, in particular when their histology confirms IgG4-related disease, can be considered as a definitive proof for type 1 AIP. For type 2, the association of IBD makes probable the diagnosis, but cannot be considered as a definitive proof.

4.5 Histology

Histology is a definitive diagnosis. Unfortunately, in the everyday clinical practice, the access to an adequately evaluable biopsy sample is not easy. Characteristic

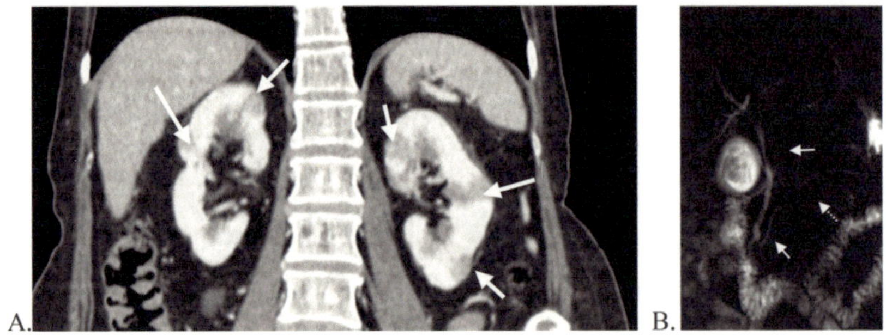

Figure 4.
(a) Nephritis in IgG4-related, type 1. AIP, concurrent with pancreatitis. Arrow: involved renal areas.
(b) Primary sclerosing cholangitis like simultaneous extra- and intrahepatic biliary tract lesions. Arrows: bile duct strictures. Pointed arrow: pancreatic duct stricture.

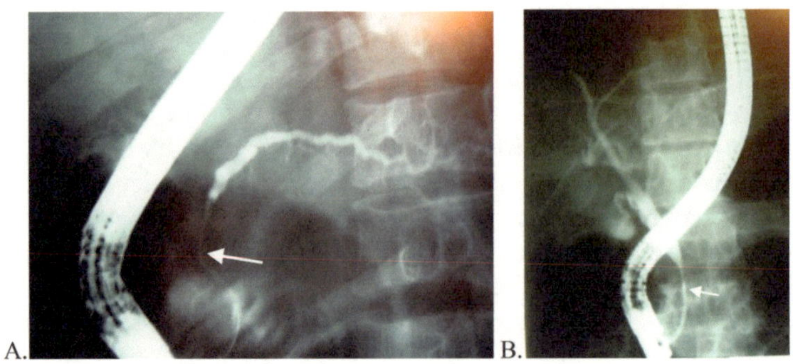

Figure 5.
ERCP of a patient. (a) Long stricture of pancreatic duct in the head (arrow), with a moderate upstream dilatation in the body and tail. (b) Bile duct stricture in the same patient (arrow).

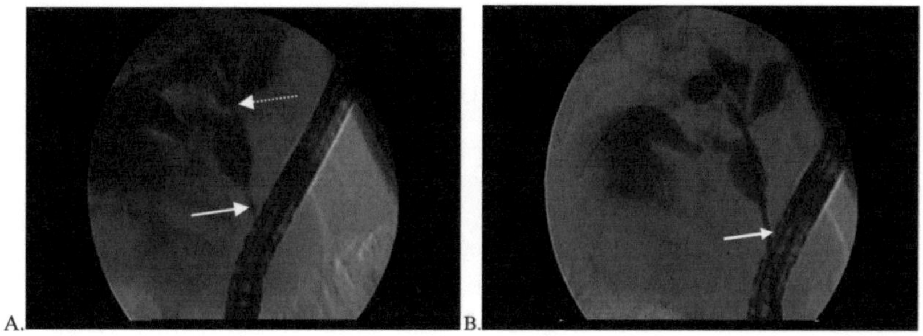

Figure 6.
ERCP of another patient. (a) Multiple stenotic segments in the bile duct: a long stricture is observed in the distal half of choledochus (arrow) and a shorter stenosis in the hepatic hilum (pointed arrow). (b) Stent (arrow) placement in the bile duct.

histology is easily seen in a surgically resected pancreas [25]. However, this is too late for the patient, who could have been treated safely with steroids instead of a major surgery. Percutaneous pancreatic biopsy made by interventional radiologists has some risks and not a currently used method. Endosonography (EUS)-guided biopsy would be the recommended way to obtain pancreatic tissue. EUS image itself is even somewhat superior to MR and gives valuable information in the differential diagnosis. In addition, fine-needle aspiration by EUS is the safest way to obtain pancreatic cytology. However, cytology has a good performance in the diagnosis of pancreatic cancer but not in the diagnosis of AIP, this latter requiring a real tissue sample biopsy [26–28].

4.5.1 When to perform EUS and FNA? Value of cytology and biopsy in differential diagnoses.

Diagnosis of type 1 AIP can be made with high certainty in many patients: clinical symptoms, characteristic images supported by elevated serum IgG4 level, and other organ involvement can assure the diagnosis without pancreatic histology. However, in the absence of these latter conditions, establishing the definitive diagnosis of even type 1 AIP can be difficult. In type 2 AIP, IgG4 is practically never increased, and IBD is the only associated pathology, but only probable diagnosis can be done without histology. With the availability of new biopsy needles (shark, core biopsy), which permit to obtain a small tissue cylinder, diagnostic performance of pancreatic biopsy has dramatically increased, without major risk of complications: clinically significant hemorrhage and pancreatitis are rare, below 1%. Thus, biopsy should be considered in every patient with a suspicion of seronegative type 1 and in type 2 AIP, preferably before initiating a relatively long steroid treatment.

4.6 Response to glucocorticosteroid treatment

The improvement in the pancreatic morphology in response to steroid treatment is very quick, easily detectable already after 2 weeks. This fact can be used even in the differential diagnosis: while AIP improves rapidly, pancreatic cancer evidently does not respond to steroids, and no change in the pancreatic morphology can be observed after 2 weeks. In addition, it was demonstrated by Moon et al. [29] that the "lost" 2 weeks did not change the resectability of the malignant lesion. This short treatment trial is only acceptable if a good biopsy is not available or the histologic finding is uncertain in a patient of high surgical risk. It means that steroid treatment trial has to be restricted to the cases, when:

- EUS and pancreatic biopsy is not available or its result is uncertain.
- Conditions of very strict and early control are assured.
- The patient is known and followed by a multidisciplinary group.
- If there is no clear improvement after 2 weeks of treatment, steroids are withdrawn and the patient goes to surgery.

In conclusion, in the everyday clinical practice, the basis of the diagnosis is radiology, showing typical characteristic images of the pancreas (**Table 2**). However, differential diagnosis is not always easy and other parameters could be of utility. Unfortunately, no specific autoantibodies have been discovered till now. Increased, >270 mg/dl serum IgG4 level seems to be quite specific but not enough sensitive in the diagnosis of type 1 AIP, and IgG4 has no value in type 2. Other organ involvement can be useful again in the diagnosis of type 1 AIP. In addition, imaging alterations do not distinguish between type 1 and type 2. Thus, type 2 AIP almost always requires biopsy and histology; in its absence the diagnosis can be only highly probable but not definitive [30]. Type 1 AIP can be definitely demonstrated without biopsy in the majority of cases. However, several patients have an undetermined AIP, which is named NOS [31], a mixture of seronegative type 1 and possible type 2 cases. A useful simple algorithm in the differential diagnosis is proposed in **Figure 7**.

After the diagnosis of AIP, the classification has practical and prognostic significance. As described above, characteristic image on MRI associated with serum IgG4 level more than double of upper limit of normal (>270 mg%) and/or simultaneous or sometimes previous presence of IgG4-related disease in other organs are sufficient to establish definitive diagnosis of type 1 AIP, even without histology. If IgG4 is normal and the only associated disease is ulcerative colitis or Crohn's disease, the classification in type 2 AIP is probable, but not definitive. If the patient does not have any associated disease, only NOS AIP is the clinically

	Increase in size	Dilatation of ducts	Parenchyma	Neighborhood
Acute pancreatitis	Diffuse	No	Edema +/− necrosis	Fluid collections
Chronic pancreatitis	Focal	Diffuse, irregular	Atrophy +/− calcifications	—
Groove pancreatitis	Head, groove	Upstream, regular	Normal	—
Autoimmune pancreatitis	Focal or diffuse	Stricture +/− slight upstream dilatation	Altered signal, contrast enhancement and diffusion	—
Pancreatic cancer	Focal (hypovascular mass)	Marked upstream	Upstream atrophy	Metastasis in lymph nodes

Note the unique combination of findings in autoimmune pancreatitis. The absence of more significant upstream dilatation of pancreatic duct and altered signal in the parenchyma, both useful as compared to pancreatic cancer. On the other hand, the absence of necrosis and peripancreatic fluid collections helps to distinguish it as compared to acute pancreatitis.

Table 2.
Characteristic alterations in pancreatic and peripancreatic morphology, useful in the differential diagnosis.

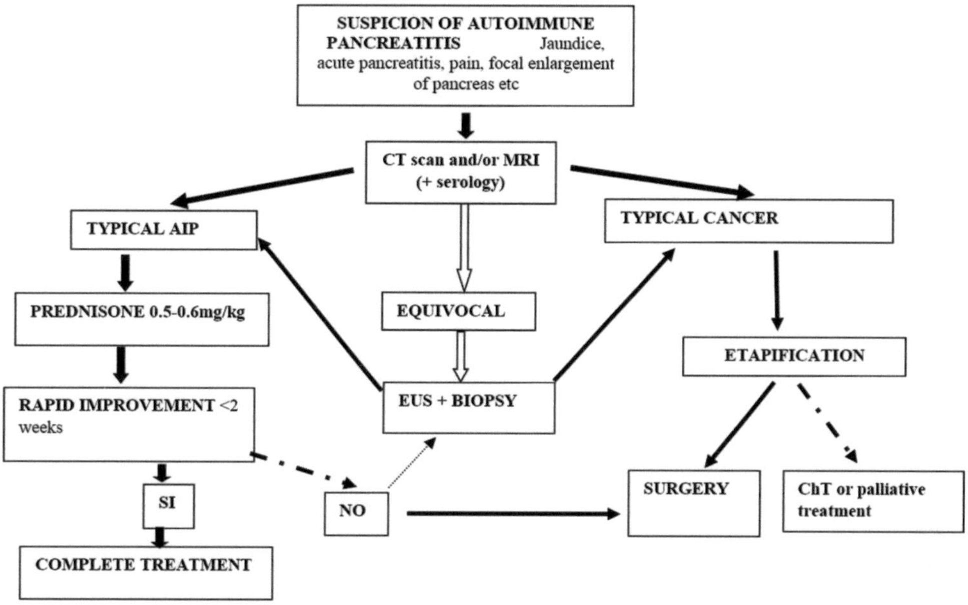

Figure 7.
A simplified algorithm for the differential diagnosis and treatment of autoimmune pancreatitis. Briefly: Once AIP is suspected on the basis of medical history or abdominal US findings, CT scan or MRI is performed, of course completed with determination of the IgG4 level in the serum. These data can be sufficient to establish definitive diagnosis of AIP or pancreatic cancer and initiate proper treatment. The effect of steroid treatment must be confirmed after a short time, about 2 weeks: if no improvement is detectable, the diagnosis of AIP is improbable, and the patients must be reevaluated for surgery or at least biopsy. If the initial workup gives an equivocal result, EUS and biopsy (not cytology!) is necessary to define the diagnosis and treatment. CT, computed tomography; MRI, magnetic resonance imaging; EUS, endosonography; Cht, chemotherapy.

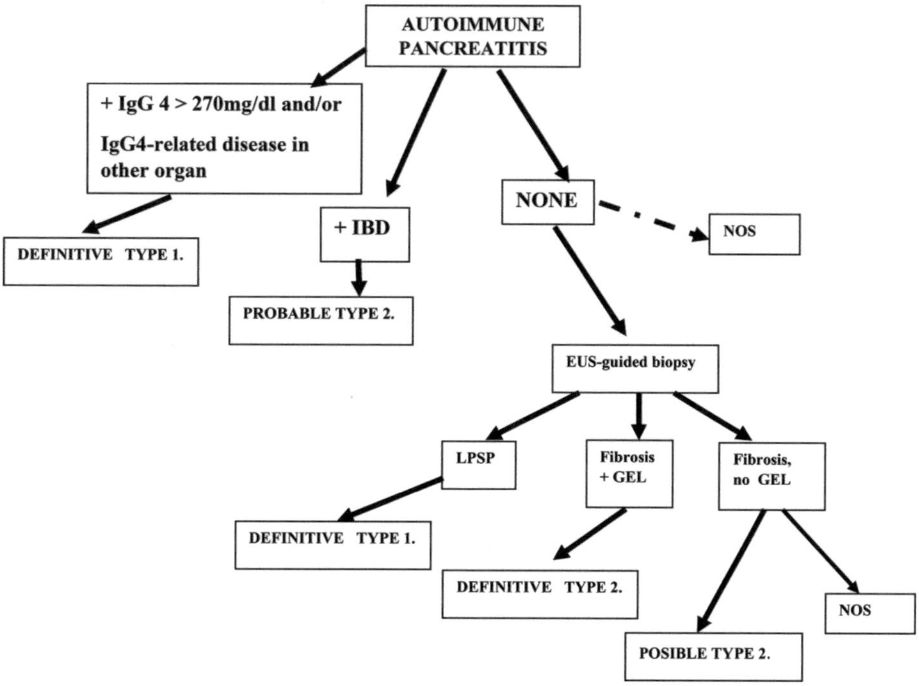

Figure 8.
Classification of AIP in different subclasses. Type 1 can be frequently demonstrated without histology, while definitive diagnosis of type 2 requires biopsy in the majority of cases. NOS is clinically a useful category, in particular, when no biopsy is available. For details, see text. LPSP, lymphoplasmacytic sclerosing pancreatitis; GEL, granulocytic epithelial lesion; NOS, Not Otherwise Specified; IBD, inflammatory bowel disease.

possible diagnosis. In these latter cases, pancreatic biopsy is advisable, guided by EUS and taking core biopsy, not cytology. Several cases will show typical histology of type 1 AIP. In others, the absence of significant IgG4-positive lymphoplasmacytic infiltration and the presence of granulocytic epithelial lesions with or without neutrophil infiltration of the pancreatic lobules prove definitively type 2 AIP. However, typical histological features of type 2 can be also absent in the core biopsy: in these cases the diagnosis continues to be NOS or sometimes probable type 2 (**Figure 8**).

5. Treatment

Once the diagnosis of AIP is established, treatment with steroids should be started. While some tendency to spontaneous improvement can exist in several cases, steroid treatment is far superior, and the recovery of pancreatic involvement is almost always complete after a relatively short, some month of treatment [32, 33]. The widely accepted dose of prednisone is relatively low, about 0.5–0.6 mg/kg/day. Others initiate the treatment with 40 mg prednisone/day. After 3–4 weeks with this treatment, the steroid dose is tapered, reducing it 5 mg/day every 2 weeks. Finally, the treatment can be stopped after the complete morphological recovery demonstrated by CT scan or magnetic resonance. However, some authors argue in favor of a maintenance treatment with prednisone in a dose as low as 5 mg/day for 2 years, and they found less recurrence with this conduct, but it is impossible to avoid completely the recurrence of the disease in the pancreas or in some other organ. The recurrent disease also responds to steroid treatment. However, in case of recurrence, it is advisable to initiate a longer treatment with some steroid-sparing agent, azathioprine (1.0–1.5 mg/kg/day) or mycophenolate (2 to 3 g/day) for several years. If these treatments fail, rituximab has been shown effective in the treatment of the first episode of the disease and also in its recurrence. In our experience, steroid treatment with or without steroid-sparing agents was effective in all but one cases; we recently used rituximab 1000 mg repeated in 15 days, i.e., 2000 mg as total dose, in one exceptional patient, with a good initial result. The Mayo Clinic experience [34] is in favor to repeat rituximab 1000 mg every 2–6 months and use it as maintenance treatment. Diabetes becomes frequently clinically overt during the acute phase, as a consequence of the disease itself and the effect of corticosteroids. Insulin treatment can be necessary, but it is transitory in the majority of the patients. Close control is mandatory in order to adjust the insulin dose, which changes rapidly during the treatment: insulin requirement initially increases and later on decreases rapidly. Clinically evident pancreatic exocrine insufficiency during the acute phase is not observed; enzyme supplementation is not necessary.

The effect of steroids is uniformly excellent. It means that if steroids fail to induce remission, one must have serious doubts in the diagnosis, whatever was the basis to establish it. In these cases histological diagnosis is mandatory and surgery is probably inevitable. In spite of the growing knowledge about AIP, the differential diagnosis can be difficult, and AIP continues to be a histological finding of some patients operated on with the suspicion of pancreatic cancer. However, surgery is not a good treatment for AIP; the recurrence without prednisone treatment continues to be a real possibility. In addition, pancreatic resection has surgical morbimortality and late metabolic consequences, which are hardly justifiable in a benign medically treatable disease.

6. Late prognosis: progression to chronic pancreatitis

AIP has been considered as a subclass of chronic pancreatitis (CP). There is no doubt that autoimmune factors can have some importance of the pathogenesis of CP and also in some cases of recurrent acute pancreatitis (RAP). There is also a possibility that the idiopathic advanced CP in several cases can be the late consequence of unrecognized and untreated AIP. However, clinical and epidemiological characteristics; morphological alterations in CT, MR, and EUS; images and histology are all quite different when compared to CP [35]. In addition, CP is a progressive damage to the pancreas, while AIP is a reversible disease after an adequate treatment. There are contradictory observations in the literature about the long-term outcome of AIP [36–38]. When we evaluate the published observations, we must be cautious, and we have to remember that AIP was definitively described only in 1995; it means that follow-up of patients for a period longer than 20 years is lacking. Biliary stenting by ERCP [39] and significant focal stenosis of the main pancreatic duct [40] were found as risk factors for formation of pancreatic stones and progression to CP. Exocrine and endocrine insufficiencies were described in a significant number of patients [41], even without detectable changes of advanced pancreatic disease. However, pancreatic enzyme replacement therapy has not been routinely used even in these cases. Our limited experiences are different: while 11 of our 74 patients had diabetes, clinically overt exocrine insufficiency was observed only in 2 of them [18], requiring oral pancreatic enzyme replacement therapy. We can find similar doubts in the literature about the risk of malignancy: higher incidence of pancreatic and extrapancreatic cancer was described by some authors [42] but not confirmed by others [43]. We did not observe malignant disease in our cohort of patients.

The possibility of AIP to PC requires longer observations. However, we insist that AIP in our opinion is not a simple subclass of CP. The differences are as strong as or even stronger than in the case of obstructive pancreatitis. Both of these entities can be reversible with an adequate timely treatment, and probably both of them can progress to CP if their cause persists unresolved [44]. If it is true, it underlines even more the importance of the early diagnosis and proper treatment.

7. Conclusions

Autoimmune pancreatitis is an increasingly recognized, relatively new disease, identified definitively only in 1995. Two types of the AIP are described, type 1 or lymphoplasmacytic sclerosing pancreatitis (LPSP) and type 2 or idiopathic duct-centric pancreatitis. While type 1 is part of an IgG4-related systemic disease, type 2 is limited to the pancreas and can be associated only with inflammatory bowel disease. The diagnosis is not easy; detection of morphological alterations is the clue in recognizing AIP and distinguishing it from other pancreatic diseases. Once the diagnosis is made, the clinical classification of types 1 and 2 also can be difficult. For this reason, an indeterminate category Not Otherwise Specified (NOS) is useful in the everyday clinical practice. All types of AIP respond rapidly and completely to steroid treatment. The late prognosis is good, but residual morphological and functional pancreatic changes can be present. Progression to advanced CP probably can be prevented with adequate treatment. These characteristics make AIP a unique pancreatic disease: its correct diagnosis avoids unnecessary surgery, and it is the only pancreatic disease when we have the possibility to achieve a complete recovery with noninvasive medical treatment. It is particular also among the autoimmune diseases: an excellent response to low-dose steroids and in relatively short time, with a real possibility to stop the treatment and a relatively low risk of recurrence or progression.

Acknowledgements

We would like to thank all the members of our group, Andrea Jiménez, Rocio Sedano, Gonzalo Cárdenas, and Fernanda Galleguillos for their contribution in the follow-up of patients and recollection of data.

Conflict of interest

The authors declare no conflict of interest.

Author details

Zoltán Berger Fleiszig[1*] and Carla Mancilla Asencio[2]

1 Gastroenterology, Department of Medicine, University of Chile's Hospital, Santiago, Chile

2 Critical Care Unit, Department of Medicine, University of Chile's Hospital, Santiago, Chile

*Address all correspondence to: zoltan@gmail.com

References

[1] Etemad B, Whitcomb DC. Chronic pancreatitis: Diagnosis, classification, and new genetic developments. Gastroenterology. 2001;**120**:682-707

[2] Chari ST. Diagnosis of autoimmune pancreatitis: The evolution of diagnostic criteria for a rare disease. Clinical Gastroenterology and Hepatology. 2017;**15**:1485-1488. DOI: 10.1016/j.cgh.2017.06.023

[3] Schneider A, Michaely H, Weiss C, Hirth M, Rückert F, Wilhelm TJ, et al. Prevalence and incidence of autoimmune pancreatitis in the population living in the Southwest of Germany. Digestion. 2017;**96**:187-198. DOI: 10.1159/000479316

[4] Nesher G, Breuer GS, Temprano K, Moore TL, Dahan D, Baer A, et al. Lupus-associated pancreatitis. Seminars in Arthritis and Rheumatism. 2006;**35**:260-267. DOI: 10.1016/j.semarthrit.2005.08.003

[5] Hernández-Molina G, Michel-Peregrina ML. Sjögren's syndrome and pancreatic affection. Reumatología Clínica. 2011;**7**:130-134. DOI: 10.1016/j.reuma.2010.07.005 (Article in Spanish)

[6] Ebert EC. Gastrointestinal and hepatic manifestations of Sjögren syndrome. Journal of Clinical Gastroenterology. 2012;**46**:25-30. DOI: 10.1097/MCG.0b013e3182329d9c

[7] Sarles H, Sarles JC, Muratore R, Guien C. Chronic inflammatory sclerosis of the pancreas–an autonomous pancreatic disease? The American Journal of Digestive Diseases. 1961;**6**:688-698

[8] Kawaguchi K. Lymphoplasmacytic sclerosing pancreatitis with cholangitis: A variant of primary sclerosing cholangitis extensively involving pancreas. Human Pathology. 1991;**22**:387-395

[9] Yoshida K, Toki F, Takeuchi T, Watanabe S, Shiratori K, Hayashi N. Chronic pancreatitis caused by an autoimmune abnormality proposal of the concept of autoimmune pancreatitis. Digestive Diseases and Sciences. 1995;**40**:1561-1568

[10] Adiga A, Nugent K. Lupus hepatitis and autoimmune hepatitis (lupoid hepatitis). The American Journal of the Medical Sciences. 2017;**353**:329-335. DOI: 10.1016/j.amjms.2016.10.014

[11] Mattoo H, Mahajan VS, Della-Torre E, Yurie Sekigami Y, Carruthers M, Wallace ZS, et al. De novo oligoclonal expansions of circulating plasmablasts in active and relapsing IgG4-related disease. The Journal of Allergy and Clinical Immunology. 2014;**134**:679-687. DOI: 10.1016/j.jaci.2014.03.034

[12] Shiokawa M, Kodama Y, Kuriyama K. Pathogenicity of IgG in patients with IgG4-related disease. Gut. 2016;**65**:1322-1332. DOI: 10.1136/gutjnl-2015-310336

[13] Ku Y, Hong SM, Fujikura K, Kim SJ, Akita M, Abe-Suzuki S, et al. IL-8 expression in granulocytic epithelial lesions of idiopathic duct-centric pancreatitis (type 2 autoimmune pancreatitis). The American Journal of Surgical Pathology. 2017;**41**:1129-1138. DOI: 10.1097/PAS.0000000000000891

[14] Aparisi L, Farre A, Gomez-Cambronero L, Martinez J, De Las Heras G, Corts J, et al. Antibodies to carbonic anhydrase and IgG4 levels in idiopathic chronic pancreatitis: Relevance for diagnosis of autoimmune pancreatitis. Gut. 2005;**54**:703-709. DOI: 10.1136/gut.2004.047142

[15] Endo T, Takizawa S, Tanaka S, Takahashi M, Fujii H, Kamisawa T, et al.

Amylase α-2A autoantibodies novel marker of autoimmune pancreatitis and fulminant type 1 diabetes. Diabetes. 2009;**58**:732-737. DOI: 10.2337/db08-0493

[16] Culver EL, Wouter LS, Evans C, Sadler R, Cargill T, Makuch M, et al. No evidence to support a role for *Helicobacter pylori* infection and plasminogen binding protein in autoimmune pancreatitis and IgG4-related disease in a UK cohort. Pancreatology. 2017;**17**:395-402. DOI: 10.1016/j.pan.2017.04.002

[17] Yu KH, Chan TM, Tsai PH, Cheng CH, Chang PY. Diagnostic performance of serum IgG4 levels in patients with IgG4-related disease. Medicine. 2015;**94**:e1707. DOI: 10.1097/MD.0000000000001707

[18] Berger Z, Jiménez A, Mancilla C, Araneda G, Sedano R. Autoimmune pancreatitis rarely progresses to advanced chronic pancreatitis—experiences from Chile. Journal of the Pancreas. 2018;**19**:244-250. Available from: http://pancreas.imedpub.com

[19] Nishimori I, Tamakoshi A, Otsuki M, The Research Committee on Intractable Diseases of the Pancreas, Ministry of Health, Labour and Welfare of Japan. Prevalence of autoimmune pancreatitis in Japan from a nationwide survey in 2002. Journal of Gastroenterology. 2007;**42**(suppl XVIII):6-8. DOI: 10.1007/s00535-007-2043-y

[20] Kanno A, Nishimori I, Masamune A, Kikuta K, Hirota M, Kuriyama S, et al. Nationwide epidemiological survey of autoimmune pancreatitis in Japan. Pancreas. 2012;**41**:835-839. DOI: 10.1097/MPA.0b013e3182480c99

[21] Kanno A, Masamune A, Okazaki K, Kamisawa T, Kawa S, Nishimori I, et al. Research committee of intractable diseases of the pancreas: Nationwide epidemiological survey of autoimmune pancreatitis in Japan in 2011. Pancreas. 2015;**44**:535-539. DOI: 10.1097/MPA.0000000000000325

[22] Sandrasegaran K, Menias CO. Imaging in autoimmune pancreatitis and immunoglobulin G4–related disease of the abdomen. Gastroenterology Clinics of North America. 2018;**47**:603-619. DOI: 10.1016/j.gtc.2018.04.007

[23] Gompertz M, Morales C, Aldana H, Castillo J, Berger Z. Cystic lesions in autoimmune pancreatitis. Case Reports in Gastroenterology. 2015;**9**:366-374. DOI: 10.1159/000441998

[24] Bi Y, Hart PA, Law R, Clain JE, Farnell MB, Gleeson FC, et al. Obstructive jaundice in autoimmune pancreatitis can be safely treated with corticosteroids alone without biliary stenting. Pancreatology. 2016;**16**: 391-396. DOI: 10.1016/j.pan.2016.03.017

[25] Zamboni G, Luttges J, Capelli P, Frulloni L, Cavallini G, Pederzoli P, et al. Histopathological features of diagnostic and clinical relevance in autoimmune pancreatitis: A study on 53 resection specimens and 9 biopsy specimens. Virchows Archiv. 2004;**445**:552-563. DOI: 10.1007/s00428-004-1140-z

[26] Deshpande V, Mino-Kenudson M, Brugge WR, Pitman MB, Fernandez-del Castillo C, Warshaw AL, et al. Endoscopic ultrasound guided fine needle aspiration biopsy of autoimmune pancreatitis: Diagnostic criteria and pitfalls. The American Journal of Surgical Pathology. 2005;**29**:1464-1471

[27] Iwashita T, Yasuda I, Doi S, Ando N, Nakashima M, Adachi S, et al. Use of samples from endoscopic ultrasound-guided19-gauge fine-needle aspiration in diagnosis of autoimmune pancreatitis. Clinical Gastroenterology

and Hepatology. 2012;**10**:316-322. DOI: 10.1016/j.cgh.2011.09.032

[28] Kanno A, Ishida K, Hamada S, Fujishima F, Unno J, Kume K, et al. Diagnosis of autoimmune pancreatitis by EUS-FNA by using a 22-gauge needle based on the international consensus diagnostic criteria. Gastrointestinal Endoscopy. 2012;**76**:594-602. DOI: 10.1016/j.gie.2012.05.014

[29] Moon SH, Kim MH, Park DH, Hwang CY, Park SJ, Lee SS, et al. Is a 2-week steroid trial after initial negative investigation for malignancy useful in differentiating autoimmune pancreatitis from pancreatic cancer? a prospective outcome study. Gut. 2008;**57**:1704-1712. DOI: 10.1136/gut.2008.150979

[30] Shimosegawa T, Chari ST, Frulloni L, Kamisawa T, Kawa S, Mino-Kenudson M, et al. International consensus diagnostic criteria for autoimmune pancreatitis: Guidelines of the international association of pancreatology. Pancreas. 2011;**40**:352-358. DOI: 10.1097/MPA.0b013e3182142fd2

[31] Ikeura T, Manfredi R, Zamboni G, Negrelli R, Capelli P, Amodio A, et al. Application of international consensus diagnostic criteria to an Italian series of autoimmune pancreatitis. United European Gastroenterology Journal. 2013;**1**:276-284. DOI: 10.1177/2050640613495196

[32] Masamune A, Nishimori I, Kikuta K, Tsuji I, Mizuno N, Iiyama T, et al. Research committee of intractable pancreas diseases in Japan: Randomised controlled trial of long-term maintenance corticosteroid therapy in patients with autoimmune pancreatitis. Gut. 2017;**66**:487-494. DOI: 10.1136/gutjnl-2016-312049

[33] Frulloni L, de Pretis N, Amodio A. Maintenance therapy in autoimmune pancreatitis: A weak light into the darkness. Annals of Translational Medicine. 2017;**5**:367. DOI: 10.21037/atm.2017.07.06

[34] Majumder S, Mohapatra S, Lennon RJ, Piovezani Ramos G, Postier N, Gleeson FC, et al. Rituximab maintenance therapy reduces rate of relapse of pancreaticobiliary immunoglobulin G4-related disease. Clinical Gastroenterology and Hepatology. 2018;**S1542-3565**(18): 30240-30244. DOI: 10.1016/j.cgh.2018.02.049

[35] Berger Z, Mancilla C. Is autoimmune pancreatitis a subclass of chronic pancreatitis? Pancreatology. 2016;**17**:55

[36] Hart P, Kamisawa T, Brugge WR, Chung JB, Culver EL, Czakó L, et al. Long-term outcomes of autoimmune pancreatitis: A multicentre, international analysis. Gut. 2013;**62**:1771-1776. DOI: 10.1136/gutjnl-2012-303617

[37] Maire F, Le Baleur Y, Rebours V, Vullierme MP, Couvelard A, Voitot H, et al. Outcome of patients with type 1 or 2 autoimmune pancreatitis. The American Journal of Gastroenterology. 2011;**106**:151-156. DOI: 10.1038/ajg.2010.314

[38] Maruyama M, Arakura N, Ozaki Y, Watanabe T, Ito T, Yoneda S, et al. Type 1 autoimmune pancreatitis can transform into chronic pancreatitis: A long-term follow-up study of 73 Japanese patients. Rheumatology International. 2013;**2013**(8):272595. DOI: 10.1155/2013/272595

[39] Matsubayashi H, Kishida Y, Iwai T, Murai K, Yoshida M, Imai K, et al. Transpapillary biliary stenting is a risk factor for pancreatic stones in patients with autoimmune pancreatitis. Endoscopy International Open. 2016;**04**:E912-E917. DOI: 10.1055/s-0042-111201

[40] Maruyama M, Arakura N, Ozaki Y, Watanabe T, Ito T, Yoneda S, et al. Risk factors for pancreatic stone formation in autoimmune pancreatitis over a long-term course. Journal of Gastroenterology. 2012;**47**:553-560. DOI: 10.1007/s00535-011-0510-y

[41] Vujasinovic M, Valente R, Maier P, von Beckerath V, Haas SL, Arnelo U, et al. Diagnosis, treatment and long-term outcome of autoimmune pancreatitis in Sweden. Pancreatology. 2018;**18**(8):900-904. DOI: 10.1016/j.pan.2018.09.003

[42] Shiokawa M, Kodama Y, Yoshimura K, Kawanami C, Mimura J, Yamashita Y, et al. Risk of cancer in patients with autoimmune pancreatitis. The American Journal of Gastroenterology. 2013;**108**:610-617. DOI: 10.1038/ajg.2012.465

[43] Hart PA, Law RJ, Dierkhising RA, Smyrk TC, Takahashi N, Chari ST. Risk of cancer in autoimmune pancreatitis: A case-control study and review of the literature. Pancreas. 2014;**43**:417-421. DOI: 10.1097/MPA.0000000000000053

[44] Takayama M, Hamano H, Ochi Y, Saegusa H, Komatsu K, Muraki T, et al. Recurrent attacks of autoimmune pancreatitis result in pancreatic stone formation. The American Journal of Gastroenterology. 2004;**99**:932-937. DOI: 10.1111/j.1572-0241.2004.04162.x